Lecture Notes in Social Networks

More information about this series at http://www.springer.com/series/8768

Arash Shaban-Nejad · John S. Brownstein
David L. Buckeridge
Editors

Public Health Intelligence and the Internet

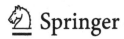 Springer

Editors
Arash Shaban-Nejad
Department of Pediatrics,
  Center for Biomedical Informatics
The University of Tennessee Health Science
  Center—Oak-Ridge National Laboratory
  (UTHSC-ORNL)
Memphis, TN
USA

David L. Buckeridge
Department of Epidemiology
  and Biostatistics and Occupational Health,
  McGill Clinical & Health Informatics
McGill University
Montreal, QC
Canada

John S. Brownstein
Department of Pediatrics, Harvard Medical
  School, Boston Children's Hospital
Harvard University
Boston, MA
USA

ISSN 2190-5428   ISSN 2190-5436   (electronic)
Lecture Notes in Social Networks
ISBN 978-3-319-88629-9   ISBN 978-3-319-68604-2   (eBook)
https://doi.org/10.1007/978-3-319-68604-2

Printed on acid-free paper

This Springer imprint is published by Springer Nature
The registered company is Springer International Publishing AG
The registered company address is: Gewerbestrasse 11, 6330 Cham, Switzerland

Preface

Severe pandemics due to highly-transmissible viruses continue to threaten the world in the twenty-first century. In a tightly interconnected world, infectious disease outbreaks can adversely affect economic growth, trade, tourism, business and industry, and social stability as well as public health. At the same time, noncommunicable diseases have become the main cause of global disability and death, imposing a crushing burden on societies and economies around the world. Public health authorities and researchers now collect data from many sources and analyze these data together to estimate the incidence and prevalence of different health conditions, as well as related risk factors. Modern surveillance systems employ tools and techniques to monitor direct and indirect signals and indicators of disease activities for early detection of outbreaks. Tracking of Internet-based health indicators complements other surveillance methods collecting data from clinical systems and registries. To provide proper alerts and timely response public health officials and researchers systematically gather news, and other reports about suspected disease outbreaks, bioterrorism, and other events of potential international public health concern, from a wide range of formal and informal sources. With the advent of modern communication technologies, many outbreak reports now originate in electronic media and electronic discussion groups. Given the ever-increasing role of the World Wide Web as a source of information in many domains including health care, accessing, managing, and analyzing its content have brought new opportunities and challenges. This is especially the case for nontraditional online resources such as social networks, blogs, news feed, twitter posts, and online communities with the sheer size and ever-increasing growth and change rate of their data. Web applications along with text processing programs are increasingly being used to harness online data and information to discover meaningful patterns identifying emerging health threats. The advances in web science and technology for data management, integration, mining, classification, filtering, and visualization have given rise to a variety of applications representing real time data on epidemics. Also, several public health surveillance tools have been recruited to use web data to detect health crises earlier than official monitoring systems. Some of the main technical and nontechnical challenges in these systems include: reliability and representativeness of the online data; redundancy and inconsistency of data; generating predictive models; timely and early detection; issues related to verification and evaluation (of the sources (number, and qualities)); and ethics, security and privacy concerns.

This book aims to highlight the latest achievements in epidemiological surveillance and Internet interventions based on monitoring online communications and interactions on the web. It presents the state of the art and the advances in the field of online disease surveillance and intervention. The edited volume contains extended and revised versions of selected papers presented at the International World Wide Web and Population Health Intelligence (W3PHI) workshop series along with some invited chapters and presents an overview of the issues, challenges, and potentials in the field, along with the new research results. The book provides information for a wide range of scientists, researchers, graduate students, industry professionals, national and international public health agencies, and NGOs interested in the theory and practice of computational models of web-based public health intelligence.

Memphis, USA   Arash Shaban-Nejad
Boston, USA   John S. Brownstein
Montreal, Canada   David L. Buckeridge

Contents

Contributors

David L. Buckeridge Department of Epidemiology & Biostatistics and Occupational Health, McGill University, Montreal, QC, Canada

Alan Chappell Pacific Northwest National Laboratory, Richland, WA, USA

Katia Charland Clinical and Health Informatics Research Group, McGill University, Montreal, QC, Canada

Lauren Charles-Smith Pacific Northwest National Laboratory, Richland, WA, USA

Soon Ae Chun City University of New York, New York, NY, USA

Courtney D. Corley Pacific Northwest National Laboratory, Richland, WA, USA

Vivek Datla Pacific Northwest National Laboratory, Richland, WA, USA

Rui Fang Research and Development, Thomson Reuters, New York City, NY, USA

James Geller New Jersey Institute of Technology, Newark, NJ, USA

Josh Harrison Pacific Northwest National Laboratory, Richland, WA, USA

Masoumeh Izadi Clinical and Health Informatics Research Group, McGill University, Montreal, QC, Canada

Xiang Ji The Bloomberg L.P., New York, NY, USA

Quanzhi Li Research and Development, Thomson Reuters, New York City, NY, USA

Xiaomo Liu Research and Development, Thomson Reuters, New York City, NY, USA

Hiroshi Mamiya Department of Epidemiology and Biostatistics and Occupational Health, McGill University, Montreal, QC, Canada

Anh Nguyen Saolasoft Inc., Centennial, CO, USA

Armineh Nourbakhsh Research and Development, Thomson Reuters, New York City, NY, USA

Umashanthi Pavalanathan Georgia Institute of Technology, Atlanta, GA, USA

Hoang Pham Piscataway, USA

Meg Pirrung Pacific Northwest National Laboratory, Richland, WA, USA

Arash Shaban-Nejad Department of Pediatrics, Center for Biomedical Informatics, University of Tennessee Health Science Center—Oak-Ridge National Lab (UTHSC-ORNL), Memphis, TN, USA

Sameena Shah Research and Development, Thomson Reuters, New York City, NY, USA

Eun Kyong Shin Department of Pediatrics, Center for Biomedical Informatics, University of Tennessee Health Science Center—Oak-Ridge National Lab (UTHSC-ORNL), Memphis, TN, USA

Tuan Tran Sullivan University, Louisville, KY, USA

Svitlana Volkova Pacific Northwest National Laboratory, Richland, WA, USA

Christopher C. Yang College of Computing and Informatics, Drexel University, Philadelphia, PA, USA

Mi Zhang College of Computing and Informatics, Drexel University, Philadelphia, PA, USA

Abbreviations

AHMM	Autoregressive Hidden Markov Models
ARMAX	Autoregressive Moving Average Exogenous Variables Model
BNs	Bayesian networks
CBOW	Continuous Bag of Words
CDC	Centers for Disease Control and Prevention
CF	Collaborative Filtering
CPT	Conditional Probability Table
DAG	Directed Acyclic Graph
DBNs	Dynamic Bayesian Networks
ED	Emergency Department
EHR	Electronic Health Records
ESMOS	Epidemic Sentiment Monitoring System
FDA	Food and Drug Administration
GOARN	Global Outbreak Alert Response Network
GPHIN	Global Public Health Intelligence Network
H7N9	Avian Influenza Type A
HIV	Human Immunodeficiency Virus
HMMs	Hidden Markov models
ICD	International Classification of Diseases
ILI	Influenza-like Illness
LDA	Latent Dirichlet Allocation
LIWC	Linguistic Inquiry and Word Count
LOD	Linked Open Data
MeSH	Medical Subject Headings
NDOS	N-dimensional order statistics
NIH	National Institutes of Health
NLM	National Library of Medicine
NLP	Natural Language Processing
NSDUH	National Survey on Drug Use and Health
PROMed-mail	The Program for Monitoring Emerging Diseases

PTSD	Post Traumatic Stress Disorder
SARS	Severe acute respiratory syndrome
SBW	Star Bright World
SHR	Social Health Records
SNS	Social Networking Services
TB	Tuberculosis
UMLS	The Unified Medical Language System Metathesaurus
UTD	User Interest and Topic Detection Model
WCA	Wavelet Coherency Analysis
WHO	World Health Organization

Public Health Intelligence and the Internet: Current State of the Art

Eun Kyong Shin and Arash Shaban-Nejad

Abstract The increasing role of Internet and the World Wide Web as a widely accessible health information source creates opportunities, along with challenges, for researchers, healthcare workers and organizations across the globe, enabling them to collect and analyze data to improving patient care, disease surveillance, and delivering online preventive or therapeutic interventions. In this chapter, after reviewing some of the applications of Internet in public health, we analyze the use of online space in clinical trials, experiments, or observations performed in clinical research, in the United States. We provide visual analytics for health data and preliminary findings from a database that systematically comprises clinical trial records. Our study focuses on clinical trial data with an "online" component in its study design. We first parse out historical trajectories of online clinical trials since its first introduction to show the use of the Internet space in health studies.

Keywords Internet intervention · Clinical trials · Social media · Population health · Surveillance · Public health

1 Introduction

The Internet has expanded the public health research beyond its traditional realm. Not only the Internet serves as effective tools for health interventions and healthcare delivery methods but also it gathers health-related data in a way that was not available before. The Internet can provide [near] real-time data and knowledge necessary for fast and timely response to public health issues. Online data can be particularly helpful in epidemic and pandemic alert and response and emergencies

E.K. Shin (✉) · A. Shaban-Nejad
Department of Pediatrics, Center for Biomedical Informatics, University of Tennessee Health Science Center—Oak-Ridge National Lab (UTHSC-ORNL), Memphis, TN, USA
e-mail: eshin3@uthsc.edu

A. Shaban-Nejad
e-mail: ashabann@uthsc.edu

© Springer International Publishing AG 2017
A. Shaban-Nejad et al. (eds.), *Public Health Intelligence and the Internet*,
Lecture Notes in Social Networks, https://doi.org/10.1007/978-3-319-68604-2_1

preparedness. In the United States, 72% of the Internet users have used the Internet for seeking health-related information whether it is directly related to themselves or for their cared ones [1]. Recent interest in social media and the use of online platforms for health research has been remarkably increased [2, 3]. There has been a wide array of application areas (e.g., epidemic detection, health intervention, discourse analysis, health education, surveillance and health promotion, etc.) and an exponentially growing use of social media analytics in health sciences [2]. Accordingly, public health practice and research made significant development using the Internet and online social media in health intervention and health surveillance.

We begin by summarizing recent studies on application of the Internet and online social media in public health and then examine the current use of the Internet in clinical trials (experiment studies or observations done in clinical research including biomedical or behavioral research studies on human participants), which are designed to answer specific questions about biomedical or behavioral interventions.

2   Digital Public Health

As with clinical applications, the digital space has been utilized in the public health field. Continuous monitoring and surveillance in public health are of critical importance and have long-established harnessing health data from healthcare facilities, which are typically resource-intensive endeavor. Digital public health has been actively explored, to partially addressing the cost and resource limitations in traditional health surveillance. In what follows, we look at some of the applications of the online public and population health intelligence.

2.1   Health Surveillance: Epidemic Detection

Digital health surveillance has been the most popular and successful area of adopting the new media. The Internet enables health professionals and the public to observe closely the most current health dynamic. Especially for detection of infectious disease dynamics, the social media serves as one of the prompt data sources that allow timely responses from health professionals and organizations at the scale beyond what traditional and formal methods have offered.

Researchers have shown that online social media data can provide a meaningful glimpse of the utmost state of infectious disease detection [4–13]. For example, influenza surveillance using online social media has attracted many attentions [4, 5]. Text mining of influenza mentions in the web environment and social media has been well correlated with actual influenza-like illness patient report data [6]. Broniatowski and his colleagues show that influenza tweet data move closely together with outpatient surveillance data provided by Centers for Disease Control and Prevention (CDC) [7]. Trajectories from online health data sources match well and are in accordance with data available from the official and traditional health-related data sources.

Online discussions are highly pertinent with what is happening in real-life and the social media has become one of the most influential mediums for health information exchange. Bernardo et al., after reviewing 32 peer-reviewed journal articles published from 2010 and 2011 using Google program for influenza surveillance, show that 66% of the studies confirm that social media health surveillance can provide compatible data to existing traditional surveillance programs [8].

Digital surveillance systems provided important early detection of numerous infectious diseases such as the outbreak of severe acute respiratory syndrome (SARS) in 2003, the influenza A (H1N1) pandemic in 2009 [9, 10], the 2013 avian influenza Type A (H7N9) outbreak in China [11, 12], and the 2010 cholera epidemic in Haiti [13]. As demonstrated in these examples, prompt and timely analysis of outbreak information alerted the healthcare organizations and public faster that official traditional outlets and active online discussions disseminated pertinent information more effectively. Broniatowski and his colleagues show that their influenza prevalence estimates are strongly correlated with those of other conventional health data providers [7]. Their system can detect the directionality of increase and decrease in influenza prevalence with 85% accuracy.

2.2 Global Health Surveillance

Infectious diseases are among major challenges of public health globally. As results of the increase in geographical ranges, from local to global, burdens of infectious disease and health surveillance have been globalized [14, 15]. Digital health surveillance can overcome geopolitical boundaries efficiently. Due to increased traffics cross borders, most cases of epidemics are less likely to be constrained within a national boundary (as evidenced in SARS 2003 [16]). Recent internationally spreading infectious diseases arose urgent needs for global health surveillance [17–19]. Domestic disease control is neither sufficient nor invincible without deterring international disease transmission. In line with this concern, World Health Organization (WHO) has launched Global Outbreak Alert Response Network (GOARN) in 2000. WHO not only pay close attention to global disease control but also active support for its technical needs [20]. Global health collaboration usually requires collective efforts from many and often distinctive entities. Digital public health is expected to be among the most efficient and cost-effective responses to the ever-growing needs for a synthesized, comprehensive global health surveillance.

Digital health surveillance system allows large-scale health surveillance with a relatively low cost. For instance, HealthMap, which is a platform for bringing together disparate data sources to achieve a unified and comprehensive view of the current global state of infectious disease, is utilizing Internet media reports [21, 22]. Flu Near You is a good example of a crowdsourced participatory epidemic monitoring system [23].

2.3 Behavior Monitoring and Sentiment Assessment

In addition, to detect disease pandemics, the new media enables the quantifying and monitoring of human behavior beyond what was possible in the past public opinion tracking at large-scale possible [24]. The Internet provides an effective platform to gauge and quantitatively measure public anxiety and concern through online social media. For example, by assessing Twitter posts or blogs, health professionals can collect and analyze quantitative and qualitative indicators to measure public anxiety about Ebola and other threatening infectious diseases [9]. Analyzing online blog posts or tweets also provides a way of measuring sentiment around any health-related event and behavior such as vaccine hesitancy [23, 25, 26].

Reviewing public data from Twitter, Salathé and Khandelwal show that sentiments about vaccination, which is a critical and effective measure in analyzing the incidence of several infectious diseases, can predicate vaccination rates in accordance with projected vaccination rates by the CDC (data came from phone survey) [27]. Running simulation models using twitter data, they also manifest how clusters of negative anti-vaccination sentiments can result in an increase in the number of unvaccinated individuals. Similarly, Mollema and colleagues scrutinized public opinion online displayed regarding measles in Netherlands [24]. Again, using Twitter data, they show that tweets are highly correlated with newly released paper articles and peaks in the online trend.

2.4 Public Health Communication

Online social media and the Internet are not only magnifying the scale but also improve the quality of public health communication. The Internet is proactively used in disseminating health-related information, both reliable and non-reliable, and delivering educational materials [2]. There is well-documented evidence showing social media and online communities are effective in disseminating health information [28–31]. Beneficial features of the digital communication are widely shared among health professionals. Physicians frequently seek and consult a wide array of social media venues and health professionals hear about the most up-to-date medical information, expose themselves to other experts, and discuss their patients with other colleagues using various online platforms [32–34]. Effective communication also connects healthcare providers and researchers with patients and public at large. In several cases, public health departments have adopted online social media as one of their primary communications tools [35].

As Eysenbach points out, digital health incorporates basic characteristics of social networking, user participation, apomediation, openness, and collaboration [3]. These factors change the way health communication is initiated and maintained. The Internet opens up a new stream of health-promoting community building, reaching further than the conventional medical institutions' scope. For example, patients regularly use social networking sites for various reasons and to find and connect with other patients and their families who are sharing similar experiences. Greene and his colleagues reviewed 15 large Facebook groups related to diabetes management and show that they provide a meaningful forum for sharing experience and getting direct feedback [36].

2.5 Health Intervention

Moving beyond gathering what is on the surface and delivering information, the Internet space has been actively explored in public health intervention. To induce desirable changes in a target population, the new media has been utilized. Online interventions are effective in changing or monitoring health-related behaviors: for example, providing an online social network community supporting smoking cessation [37], encouraging HIV testing through text messages [38] and using Facebook to promote HIV prevention [39]. Also by investigating ten published media intervention studies (eight papers using web-based, one with mobile phones and one on SNS) related to adolescent sexual health, Kylene and colleagues reported that they were all successful (i.e., in delaying first intercourse, condom use etc.) [40]. Likewise, Mock and his colleagues show that a web-based education for cancer screening is effective [41]. In their studies, participants in the media intervention group showed a relatively significant increased cancer testing rate from 70.1 to 75.5%.

The applications of digital health for behavioral change cover a wide range of topics from sexual health to mental health. Certainly, web-based interventions are different from in-person health interventions. On the one hand, geographical accessibility to patients and public is greater than traditional in-person interventions. Its cost-effectiveness for large-scale intervention is laudable compared to the traditional method. On the other, the sampling process requires further carefulness to overcome the skewed user population and the privacy issue needs to be considered seriously. Therefore, target specification and scope conditions are critical for successful Internet-based health interventions [42].

3   Online Clinical Trials

Along with the increased interest in digital health surveillance, the number of clinical studies with online components has been increased.[1] To trace how the recent clinical trials, harness the Internet, a dataset comprising 1563 clinical studies referencing "Online" from ClinicalTrials.gov was downloaded on Nov 3, 2016.[2] The website is maintained by the National Library of Medicine (NLM) at the National Institutes of Health (NIH) providing information on both publicly and privately supported clinical trials in the United States. The registry begins usually when a clinical study begins and is updated throughout the trial process. There is a total of 1563 clinical trials implementing online globally and 798 cases of them are focusing on the U.S. With a focus on the clinical trials in the U.S., we first parse out the historical trajectories of online clinical trials since its first introduction.

3.1   Historical Trajectory of Online Clinical Trials

According to ClinicalTrials.gov, the first U.S. focused clinical trial with "online" elements was conducted in 1999. The first study in the U.S. recorded from the database exhibits their rationales as following: "This study seeks to evaluate the impact of Star Bright World (SBW) on hospitalized children. SBW is a virtual environment designed to link seriously ill children into an interactive online community where they can play games, learn about their condition, or talk with other ill children who are connected to the network. Our outcome evaluation of SBW will include assessments of pain, mood (anxious, depressed and energetic), anger, loneliness, and willingness to return to the NIH for the treatment of children who are being treated at NIH. They will be assessed while engaging in "normal" recreational activities (in one of two available playrooms) and while using SBW. In addition, we will conduct a process evaluation of the implementation of SBW [43]."

Based on this description, one can see that the early idea of application of the digital space is well reflected in the study design. Since then the implementation of online space for clinical research has been dramatically grown as shown in Fig. 1. We present the total number of newly registered clinical trials for each year. It has been widely increased in its number of studies (projects and papers) and along with the subject field has been diversified. Figure 1 compares the clinical trials at the clinical trials globally, which is the total number of online clinical trials, and those focusing only on the United States. From the diagrams, we can see that most of the online clinical trials are based in the U.S.

---

[1]A clinical trial is a study where individuals voluntarily participate health-related scientific research and are assigned to interventions and then evaluated for effects on health-related outcomes.

[2]ClinicalTrial.gov was conceived as a result of the Food and Drug Administration (FDA) Modernization Act of 1997 and launched by NIH and FDA 2000.

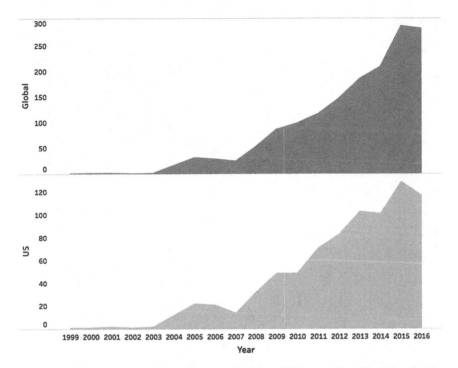

Fig. 1 Historical trajectories of online clinical trial. *Notes* All accumulative trajectories of online clinical trials are presented in the top part. The bottom graph represents online clinical trials focusing on the U.S. *Data source* ClinicalTrials.gov

Clinical trials can be divided into two major categories, interventional and observational. According to Clinicaltrial.gov, the first type, an interventional trial, is the case of participating patients received one or more intervention to gauge the effects of the interventions on biomedical or health-related outcomes. Observational studies are performed when investigators evaluate health outcomes of participants according to their routine medical care. Patients may have been received interventional treatment, independent of researchers' intention. The recent increase in the number of online clinical trials is mostly driven by the increased popularity of interventional studies. As shown in Fig. 2, interventional trials using online space exponentially increased since the first introduction in 2001 although the number of observational studies has been steadily increased as well.

3.2 Diversification of Online Clinical Trials

Figure 3 presents the historical trajectory of diversification of applied health conditions mentioned in the clinical trials. This graph shows that the number of online

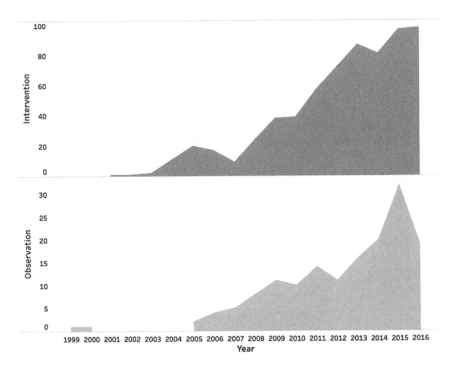

Fig. 2 Interventional versus observational online clinical trials. *Notes* The top graph shows accumulative interventional online clinical trials. The bottom graph represents observational online clinical trials. *Data source* ClinicalTrials.gov

clinical trials has been increased not only in quantity but also in diversity. Each color represents a unique health condition that has been targeted through online clinical trials in each year. A wide variety of application areas (i.e., epidemic detection, health intervention, discourse analysis, and health education) have been explored in the online clinical trials.

The most commonly targeted health conditions are cancer (68 cases, comprises all cancer types except breast cancer), obesity (64 cases), depression (34 cases), smoking (32 cases), HIV (26 cases), diabetes (25 cases), breast cancer (22 cases), and health-related behaviors (22 cases).[3] These most commonly visited health conditions show the pertinent arena where the Internet is more relevant. Due to the importance of focusing on the modifiable risk factors in preventing chronic diseases, we found out that recent online clinical trials tend to focus more on behavioral changes. For example, most of the cancer trials are focusing on online

---

[3]We use the condition variables as they provided from ClinicalTrials.gov. Although they could be debatable, we used the self-reported classifications. Investigators report their own classification of applied health conditions. For example, under the health-related behavior category, we can find physical activity promotion intervention, personal medication records management, and eating habit monitoring.

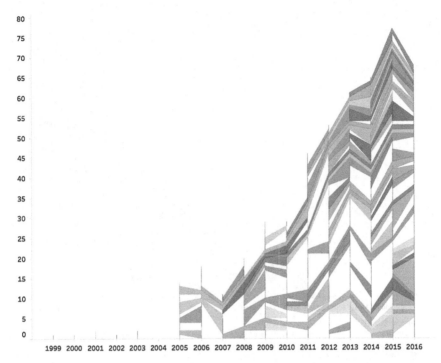

Fig. 3 Diversification of applied health conditions. *Notes* Each color represents a specific health condition. Due to limited page space, the color index is not included in this figure. *Data source* ClinicalTrials.gov

support network systems and how the online support can improve the patients' conditions and ease the pain of getting through the ups and downs. Online clinical trials exhibit a strong affinity for health interventions that require close and constant monitoring of behavioral patterns of the patients. For example, most of the trials focusing on health conditions such as obesity, depression, and smoking directly track and monitor health behavior of participants.

Not only the health conditions in clinical trials have been diversified within the past recent years, but also sponsoring funding sources have expanded, which shows a growing general interest in Internet applications in health research and practice. Figure 4 presents the historical changes in compositions of funding sources for the clinical trials that are included in our study. This variable describes which kind of organizations provides support (e.g., providing facilities, expertise, or financial resources) for the study.

According to ClinicalTrials.gov, the types of funder are broadly categorized as follows: National Institutes of Health (NIH), other U.S. Federal agencies (e.g., the Food and Drug Administration, Centers for Disease Control and Prevention (CDC), the U.S. Department of Veterans Affairs), industries (pharmaceutical and device companies), and all others (including individuals, universities, and community-based

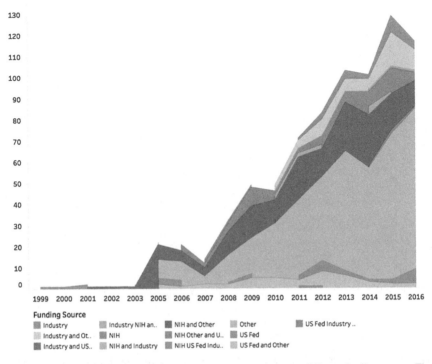

Fig. 4 Funding source information. *Notes* Each color represents a different funding source. The total numbers are shown as accumulative. *Data source* ClinicalTrials.gov

organizations). Additionally, multi-agents funded studies are marked by the combination of the funders. If a study is partially funded by NIH and a university, the funding type category is assigned to NIH and Other.

As shown in Fig. 4, at its early stage, the National Institute of Health (NIH) was the main source of funding for online clinical trials. Then other types of funding sources became available, independently or in collaboration with NIH. The industry also has grown to become an important sponsoring sector. Moreover, other U.S. Federal agencies started to provide funding since 2005 and they have remained a steady source, although with a limited quantity. Diversification of funding sources may well reflect the increased interest in the use of online methods in health applications.

3.3 *Funding Sources and Disease Networks*

Next, we take a closer look on who funds what kind of health research through applying social network presentation. Figure 5a shows the two-mode network

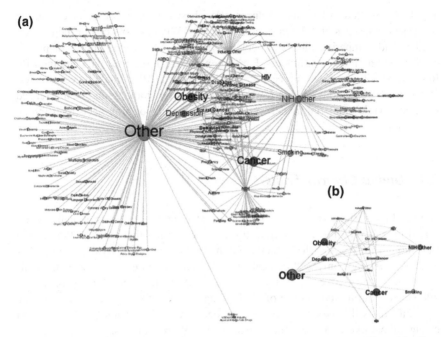

Fig. 5 Funding sources and disease networks. *Notes* Red nodes represent different funding sources. The node "other" represents federal agencies other than NIH. Green nodes represent health conditions for which online clinical trials applied. *Data source* ClinicalTrials.gov

(global network) of Health Conditions and Funding Sources. Each circle (node) in Fig. 5 represents either a health condition or a funding source. The green nodes are health conditions that online clinical trials have been applied for and the red nodes are funding agents who provide funding for the projects focusing on the health conditions.[4] Ties (lines between nodes) in the graph represent the funding relations between the health conditions and the funding agents. Additionally, the size of nodes, which indicates betweenness centrality, shows relative connectivity and centrality in the network. From the network, we found out that the major funding sources for online clinical trials mostly come from the funding sources other than NIH, other U.S. Federal agencies or Industry.

Network density, which is measured by the total number of existing ties divided by the total number of possible ties given the number of nodes in a given network, is low (0.024), which indicates that there is heterogeneity in connectivity reflecting diverse health conditions under investigation.

In Fig. 5b, we highlighted the funding networks for the major health conditions namely cancer, obesity, depression, smoking, HIV, diabetes, breast cancer, stress,

---

[4]As discussed earlier, we use the condition categories that are reported by investigators of the online clinical trials.

and health-related behaviors.[5] Cancer and obesity have most diverse funding sources (seven types of different funding agents).[6] When we switch our focus to the funders and comparing their ego network, we can identify the patterns of preferences of different types of funders. For example, we can see both NIH and industry funders heavily invested in cancer and obesity-related online clinical studies. However, NIH is more leaning towards researches on smoking and health-related behaviors while industrial funders seem to be more in favor of projects focusing on depression and breast cancer.

3.4 Digital Clinical Trials

Online clinical trials are much bigger in their sizes compared to traditional studies. Based on our preliminary research, however, we found that most of the clinical trials do not fully utilize the capacity and the services provided by the Internet. For example, there are only 122 clinical trials that recruit more than 1000 individuals and there are only 25 cases that are using 10,000 and more enrollment size out of 798 studies. Furthermore, most of the funding goes to chronic diseases in compare with infectious diseases. Additionally, funders invested thoroughly on behavioral change, most likely to target the related modifiable risk factors.

There are also a few limitations of the empirical investigation of digital clinical trials (see Zarin et al. [44] and Califf et al. [45] for further analysis). Not all the clinical trials conducted in the U.S., are reported to the ClinicalTrials.gov. By Food and Drug Administration Amendments Act of 2007 (FDAAA, specifically section 801) requirements, some studies without involving any drug, biologic, or device are not required by law to report. Although voluntary registration of those exceptions has been increased, they fall outside the scope of the present study. This limitation may lead to underestimating the current state by only looking at those reported to NIH. Therefore, the results must be interpreted and generalized with caution.

4 Remaining Issues in Digital Public Health Intelligence

Premises of digital public health shine not without some remaining issues. Observational data obtained from online resources are not designed to be fully representative of a target population. There are ethical challenges as well as legal

---

[5]Again, the categorization may appear controversial. The chronical disease category includes studies as "Does Access to an EHR Patient Portal Influence Chronic Disease Outcomes? Dyspnea Self-Management: Internet or Face-to-Face." We used their own self-classifications that are available from the data source.

[6]Here, we count different combination of funding sources as one independent type of funding.

consideration, security, and privacy issues. There are also many challenges regarding integration and analytic aspects of online social media and health data. Online social media data differs from traditional data sources in several ways.

First, the coexistence of anonymous and identifiable users may question the reliability and the quality of the data [46]. This problem may lead to a more serious situation because many people search information online even before they talk with medical or health professionals [47].

As anyone can contribute to the online health discourse, the reliability of some information has to be processed with caution. For instance, Greene and his college warn for the quality control in online health-related groups [36]. They found that promotional activities are not filtered. For example, marketing agents can disguise their identities as patients and upload advertisements as a true experience. Additionally, online communities are vulnerable to personal data collection. Patients may share their personal medical information that can be used for other marketing purposes. Therefore, continuous efforts from health professionals and the public need to be alert to any anonymous mal-information which can be excelling the reliable medical information.

Moreover, the effectiveness of the social media intervention is harder to measure [48, 49]. Unstructured large datasets from the Internet tend to be not suitable to make a causal argument and are limited in its capability of sorting out confounding factors [50]. Dennison and her colleagues expressed similar concerns [51]. Experiments using a health behavior monitoring app, they acknowledged the limitation of assuring positive effects between web-based devices and behavioral changes.

Additionally, uneven digital development (across different geographical locations) needs further attention. The distribution and circulation of health-related information on the Internet are not evenly distributed worldwide [17]. The global spread of infectious disease is being observed more frequently [52]. Given that health problems are no longer confined to specific regions, the regional digital disparity is not a dismissible issue. Alleviated geographical digital disparity will warrant more efficient global health surveillance.

Recently, the tendency of the health-related text analysis reflects the differences in the usage patterns of the population on the Internet. Paul and his colleagues highlight urgent attentions on how to use a short hashtag or tweet to make a meaningful warning system or a large systematic analysis [53].

5 Conclusion

In this chapter, we explored the potential use of online platforms in public and population health for health surveillance, behavior monitoring and sentiment assessment, health intervention, public health communication and promotion. We then studied the use of the Internet in clinical trials in the United States. Despite aforementioned limitations, expected and earned benefits are much to be applauded and worth for further investment. Cost-effectiveness, increased reachability, promptness are some of the common benefits of exploiting the Internet for health intervention [29]. Also, online social media can provide personalized and well-tailored health information in a timely manner [54].

Utilizing audience networks to disseminate and share health information lead to broader and diverse population at reach beyond the magnitude the traditional method can offer [54]. According to the Health tracking survey 2012, the disparity in accessibility to the Internet has been dramatically decreased and 81% of the U.S. adults use the Internet and when it comes to health-related Internet exploration, racial differences are smaller than general Internet users [1, 55]. One may argue that demographic characteristics of Internet users are skewed toward the younger generation. Particularly, the age-driven preference across different types of social media with which they frequent hinder researchers garner representative samples if they only focus on a limited number of Internet platforms. Younger generations search health information online more actively than older generations [1]. However, health concerned individuals are often nested in larger family and friend networks. For example, one may not actively engage with social media, but her or his family members and friends may. Therefore, nonactive users are not completely immune to what is discussed and delivered online.

Online environment also broadens the communication channels between health providers/researchers and patients/public by facilitating multi-way communications and encourages public engagement [54]. Moreover, the information in the scientific journal articles, which traditionally circulated through limited channels, can be widely shared, distributed, and cited through Facebook pages, Blogs, and Twitter posts. The very feature enables participatory epidemiology [19]. Most importantly, the digital health surveillance enables real-time data collection, providing [near] real-time data and knowledge necessary for fast and timely response to public health issues, especially in epidemic and pandemic alert and response and emergencies preparedness. Hence, digital health surveillance is expected to enhance specificity and sensitivity in public health [8]. In addition, digital health technologies enable health professionals at global level to collect and monitor health data with lower cost and localized service delivery as well.

References

1. Fox, S., Duggan, M.: Health Online 2013. Pew Internet & American Life Project, Washington, DC (2013)
2. Moorhead, S.A., Hazlett, D.E., Harrison, L., Carroll, J.K., Irwin, A., Hoving, C.: A new dimension of health care: systematic review of the uses, benefits, and limitations of social media for health communication. J. Med. Internet Res. **15**(4) (2013)
3. Eysenbach, G.: Medicine 2.0: social networking, collaboration, participation, apomediation, and openness. J. Med. Internet Res. **10**(3), e22 (2008)
4. Lampos, V., Cristianini, N.: Tracking the flu pandemic by monitoring the social web. In: 2010 2nd International Workshop on Cognitive Information Processing (CIP), pp. 411–416. IEEE (2010)

5. Culotta, A.: Towards detecting influenza epidemics by analyzing Twitter messages. In: Proceedings of the First Workshop on Social Media Analytics, pp. 115–122. ACM (2010)
6. Corley, C.D., Cook, D.J., Mikler, A.R., Singh, K.P.: Text and structural data mining of influenza mentions in web and social media. Int. J. Environ. Res. Public health **7**(2), 596–615 (2010)
7. Broniatowski, D.A., Paul, M.J., Dredze, M.: National and local influenza surveillance through Twitter: an analysis of the 2012–2013 influenza epidemic. PLoS ONE **8**(12), e83672 (2013)
8. Bernardo, T.M., Rajic, A., Young, I., Robiadek, K., Pham, M.T., Funk, J.A.: Scoping review on search queries and social media for disease surveillance: a chronology of innovation. J. Med. Internet Res. **15**(7), e147 (2013)
9. Chun-Hai Fung, I., Wong, K.: Efficient use of social media during the avian influenza A (H7N9) emergency response. West. Pac. Surveill. Response J. **4**(4), 1 (2013)
10. Salathé, M., Freifeld, C.C., Mekaru, S.R., Tomasulo, A.F., Brownstein, J.S.: Influenza A (H7N9) and the importance of digital epidemiology. N. Engl. J. Med. **369**(5), 401 (2013)
11. Zhang, E.X., Yang, Y., Di Shang, R., Simons, J.J.P., Quek, B.K., Yin, X.F., See, W., Oh, O. S.H., Nandar, K.S.T., Ling, V.R.Y.: Leveraging social networking sites for disease surveillance and public sensing: the case of the 2013 avian influenza A (H7N9) outbreak in China. West. Pac. Surveill. Response J. **6**(2), 66–72 (2015)
12. Gu, H., Chen, B., Zhu, H., Jiang, T., Wang, X., Chen, L., Jiang, Z., Zheng, D., Jiang, J.: Importance of Internet surveillance in public health emergency control and prevention: evidence from a digital epidemiologic study during avian influenza A H7N9 outbreaks. J. Med. Internet Res. **16**(1), e20 (2014)
13. Chunara, R., Andrews, J.R., Brownstein, J.S.: Social and news media enable estimation of epidemiological patterns early in the 2010 Haitian cholera outbreak. Am. J. Trop. Med. Hyg. **86**(1), 39–45 (2012)
14. Morse, S.S.: Factors in the emergence of infectious diseases. In: Plagues and Politics, pp. 8–26. Springer (2001)
15. Morens, D.M., Folkers, G.K., Fauci, A.S.: The challenge of emerging and re-emerging infectious diseases. Nature **430**(6996), 242–249 (2004)
16. Heymann, D.L.: The international response to the outbreak of SARS in 2003. Philos. Trans. R. Soc. B Biol. Sci. **359**(1447), 1127 (2004)
17. Chan, E.H., Brewer, T.F., Madoff, L.C., Pollack, M.P., Sonricker, A.L., Keller, M., Freifeld, C.C., Blench, M., Mawudeku, A., Brownstein, J.S.: Global capacity for emerging infectious disease detection. Proc. Natl. Acad. Sci. **107**(50), 21701–21706 (2010)
18. Binder, S., Levitt, A.M., Sacks, J.J., Hughes, J.M.: Emerging infectious diseases: public health issues for the 21st century. Science **284**(5418), 1311–1313 (1999)
19. Hartley, D.M.: Using social media and internet data for public health surveillance: the importance of talking. Milbank Q. **92**(1), 34–39 (2014)
20. WHO: The world health report 2007: a safer future: global public health security in the 21st century (2007)
21. Brownstein, J., Freifeld, C.: HealthMap: the development of automated real-time internet surveillance for epidemic intelligence. Euro. Surveill. **12**(11), E071129 (2007)
22. Freifeld, C.C., Mandl, K.D., Reis, B.Y., Brownstein, J.S.: HealthMap: global infectious disease monitoring through automated classification and visualization of Internet media reports. J. Am. Med. Inform. Assoc. **15**(2), 150–157 (2008)
23. Smolinski, M.S., Crawley, A.W., Baltrusaitis, K., Chunara, R., Olsen, J.M., Wójcik, O., Santillana, M., Nguyen, A., Brownstein, J.S.: Flu near you: crowdsourced symptom reporting spanning 2 influenza seasons. Am. J. Public Health **105**(10), 2124–2130 (2015)
24. Mollema, L., Harmsen, I.A., Broekhuizen, E., Clijnk, R., De Melker, H., Paulussen, T., Kok, G., Ruiter, R., Das, E.: Disease detection or public opinion reflection? Content analysis of tweets, other social media, and online newspapers during the measles outbreak in The Netherlands in 2013. J. Med. Internet Res. **17**(5) (2015)

25. Leaman, R., Wojtulewicz, L., Sullivan, R., Skariah, A., Yang, J., Gonzalez, G.: Towards internet-age pharmacovigilance: extracting adverse drug reactions from user posts to health-related social networks. In: Proceedings of the 2010 Workshop on Biomedical Natural Language Processing, pp. 117–125. Association for Computational Linguistics (2010)
26. Brien, S., Naderi, N., Shaban-Nejad, A., Mondor, L., Kroemker, D., Buckeridge, D.L.: Vaccine attitude surveillance using semantic analysis: constructing a semantically annotated corpus. In: Proceedings of the 22nd International Conference on World Wide Web, pp. 683–686. ACM, Rio de Janeiro, Brazil (2013)
27. Salathé, M., Khandelwal, S.: Assessing vaccination sentiments with online social media: implications for infectious disease dynamics and control. PLoS Comput. Biol. 7(10), e1002199 (2011)
28. Griffiths, F., Cave, J., Boardman, F., Ren, J., Pawlikowska, T., Ball, R., Clarke, A., Cohen, A.: Social networks—the future for health care delivery. Soc. Sci. Med. 75(12), 2233–2241 (2012)
29. Griffiths, F., Lindenmeyer, A., Powell, J., Lowe, P., Thorogood, M.: Why are health care interventions delivered over the internet? A systematic review of the published literature. J. Med. Internet Res. 8(2), e10 (2006)
30. Scanfeld, D., Scanfeld, V., Larson, E.L.: Dissemination of health information through social networks: Twitter and antibiotics. Am. J. Infect. Control 38(3), 182–188 (2010)
31. Capurro, D., Cole, K., Echavarría, M.I., Joe, J., Neogi, T., Turner, A.M.: The use of social networking sites for public health practice and research: a systematic review. J. Med. Internet Res. 16(3), e79 (2014)
32. Courtney, K.: The use of social media in healthcare: organizational, clinical, and patient perspectives. Enabling Health and Healthcare through ICT: Available, Tailored and Closer 183, 244 (2013)
33. Thompson, L.A., Black, E., Duff, W.P., Black, N.P., Saliba, H., Dawson, K.: Protected health information on social networking sites: ethical and legal considerations. J. Med. Internet Res. 13(1), e8 (2011)
34. Cooper, C.P., Gelb, C.A., Rim, S.H., Hawkins, N.A., Rodriguez, J.L., Polonec, L.: Physicians who use social media and other internet-based communication technologies. J. Am. Med. Inform. Assoc. 19(6), 960–964 (2012)
35. Thackeray, R., Neiger, B.L., Smith, A.K., Van Wagenen, S.B.: Adoption and use of social media among public health departments. BMC Public Health 12(1), 242 (2012)
36. Greene, J.A., Choudhry, N.K., Kilabuk, E., Shrank, W.H.: Online social networking by patients with diabetes: a qualitative evaluation of communication with Facebook. J. Gen. Intern. Med. 26(3), 287–292 (2011)
37. Cobb, N.K., Graham, A.L., Abrams, D.B.: Social network structure of a large online community for smoking cessation. Am. J. Public Health 100(7), 1282–1289 (2010)
38. Déglise, C., Suggs, L.S., Odermatt, P.: Short message service (SMS) applications for disease prevention in developing countries. J. Med. Internet Res. 14(1), e3 (2012)
39. Jaganath, D., Gill, H.K., Cohen, A.C., Young, S.D.: Harnessing Online Peer Education (HOPE): integrating C-POL and social media to train peer leaders in HIV prevention. AIDS Care 24(5), 593–600 (2012)
40. Guse, K., Levine, D., Martins, S., Lira, A., Gaarde, J., Westmorland, W., Gilliam, M.: Interventions using new digital media to improve adolescent sexual health: a systematic review. J. Adolesc. Health 51(6), 535–543 (2012)
41. Mock, J., McPhee, S.J., Nguyen, T., Wong, C., Doan, H., Lai, K.Q., Nguyen, K.H., Nguyen, T.T., Bui-Tong, N.: Effective lay health worker outreach and media-based education for promoting cervical cancer screening among Vietnamese American women. Am. J. Public Health 97(9), 1693–1700 (2007)
42. Horvath, K.J., Ecklund, A.M., Hunt, S.L., Nelson, T.F., Toomey, T.L.: Developing Internet-based health interventions: a guide for public health researchers and practitioners. J. Med. Internet Res. 17(1), e28 (2015)

43. Brokstein, R.T., Cohen, S.O., Walco, G.A.: STARBRIGHT World and psychological adjustment in children with cancer: a clinical series. Child. Health Care **31**(1), 29–45 (2002)
44. Zarin, D.A., Tse, T., Williams, R.J., Califf, R.M., Ide, N.C.: The ClinicalTrials.gov results database—update and key issues. N. Engl. J. Med. **2011**(364), 852–860 (2011)
45. Califf, R.M., Zarin, D.A., Kramer, J.M., Sherman, R.E., Aberle, L.H., Tasneem, A.: Characteristics of clinical trials registered in ClinicalTrials.gov, 2007–2010. JAMA **307**(17), 1838–1847 (2012)
46. Ventola, C.L.: Social media and health care professionals: benefits, risks, and best practices. Pharm. Ther. **39**(7), 491 (2014)
47. Hesse, B.W., Nelson, D.E., Kreps, G.L., Croyle, R.T., Arora, N.K., Rimer, B.K., Viswanath, K.: Trust and sources of health information: the impact of the Internet and its implications for health care providers: findings from the first Health Information National Trends Survey. Arch. Intern. Med. **165**(22), 2618–2624 (2005)
48. Korda, H., Itani, Z.: Harnessing social media for health promotion and behavior change. Health Promot. Pract. **14**(1), 15–23 (2013)
49. Velasco, E., Agheneza, T., Denecke, K., Kirchner, G., Eckmanns, T.: Social media and internet-based data in global systems for public health surveillance: a systematic review. Milbank Q. **92**(1), 7–33 (2014)
50. Fung, I.C.-H., Tse, Z.T.H., Fu, K.-W.: The use of social media in public health surveillance. West. Pac. Surveill. Response J. **6**(2), 3–6 (2015)
51. Dennison, L., Morrison, L., Conway, G., Yardley, L.: Opportunities and challenges for smartphone applications in supporting health behavior change: qualitative study. J. Med. Internet Res. **15**(4), e86 (2013)
52. Mathers, C., Fat, D.M., Boerma, J.T.: The Global Burden of Disease: 2004 Update. World Health Organization (2008)
53. Paul, M.J., Sarker, A., Brownstein, J.S., Nikfarjam, A., Scotch, M., Smith, K.L., Gonzalez, G.: Social media mining for public health monitoring and surveillance. In: Pacific Symposium on Biocomputing (PSB), pp. 468–479 (2016)
54. Center for Disease Control and Prevention: The Health Communicator's Social Media Toolkit. Atlanta, GA (2011)
55. Fox, S., Jones, S.: The Social Life of Health Information: Americans' Pursuit of Health Takes Place Within a Widening Network of Both Online and Offline Sources. Pew Internet & American Life Project Google Scholar, Washington, DC (2010)

Social Health Records: Gaining Insights into Public Health Behaviors, Emotions, and Disease Trajectories

Soon Ae Chun, James Geller and Xiang Ji

Abstract Social media and personal health monitoring devices (e.g., Fitbit) provide abundant patient-generated health-related data. These open health data, generated via patient engagement and sharing, are referred to as *Social Health Records* (*SHR*) as opposed to the EHR (Electronic Health Records) that are created and entered by clinicians. SHRs are changing the healthcare paradigm from the authoritative provider-centric model to a collaborative and patient-oriented healthcare framework. This chapter proposes an *SHR Integration and Analytics Framework* to leverage Social Health Records for gaining insights into population-level and individual-level healthcare practices and behaviors, as well as emotions. The framework defines a pipeline for generating knowledge from the social health data sources to the end users, including the patients themselves, public health officials, and healthcare providers. The SHR integration and analytics framework build a coherent knowledge base, linking the Social Health Records that are "spilled" in distributed online social media, with other online health information sources, such as results from authoritative medical research. The semantic integration model of heterogeneous health data sources provides population-level health analytics and reasoning capabilities to gain intelligence on public healthcare issues and practices. The SHR is shown to be a valuable resource for epidemic surveillance systems with real-time monitoring. We focus on an approach to quantifying the SHR-based public emotions for measuring health concern levels and for tracking them, and propose SHR-based predictive models to infer individual-level and population-level comorbidity predictions and comorbidity progression trajectories.

S.A. Chun (✉)
City University of New York, New York, NY, USA
e-mail: Soon.Chun@csi.cuny.edu

J. Geller
New Jersey Institute of Technology, Newark, NJ, USA
e-mail: james.geller@njit.edu

X. Ji
The Bloomberg L.P., New York, NY, USA

© Springer International Publishing AG 2017
A. Shaban-Nejad et al. (eds.), *Public Health Intelligence and the Internet*,
Lecture Notes in Social Networks, https://doi.org/10.1007/978-3-319-68604-2_2

Keywords Social Health Records (SHR) · Social media analytics · Social media content mining · Public health monitoring · Semantic integration · Social health knowledge base · Linked health data

1 Introduction

There is a large amount of health information available for any patient to address his/her health concerns. The freely available health datasets include open government health datasets, at the national, state or community level, such as OpenHealthdata.gov ranging from Medicare data to epidemiology; Web health resources curated by experts such as WebMD; and the personal health records shared by the patients on open or registered online social media services such as PatientsLikeMe. These are so-called *open health data*, which are readily accessible and downloadable. The patient-generated and shared data include the conditions, treatments, side effects, health histories, and personal physical, psychological, emotional and relationship experiences of individual patients. This data resembles the Electronic Health Record (EHR), which is defined as an electronic version of a patient's medical history that is collected and maintained by the provider (e.g., clinicians) over time.

The EHR system allows capturing the key administrative and clinical data relevant to that person's care, including demographics, progress notes, problems, medications, vital signs, past medical history, immunizations, laboratory data, and radiology reports. Since the open online health records shared by patients or family care givers capture similar data about the patients, we call this *Social Health Record* (*SHR*) to distinguish from the closed EHR. Some of the key characteristics of EHR and SHR are shown in Table 1.

The SHR is capturing many instances of personal healthcare experiences, practices and other health-related behaviors, while the EHR is capturing the clinical data necessary to provide care. Even though a doctor prescribes a medicine X, the patient may consume a substitute medicine Y. The intention of sharing the Social Health Records is support-oriented with information and experience sharing, while the EHR is primarily care-oriented to address the conditions. The SHR expresses emotional and psychological attitudes, opinions and comments in ordinary language riddled with ambiguities, while the EHR may capture mostly the factual statements in expert language to avoid vagueness or ambiguities. Another difference is that the EHR is hard to share, protected by the HIPAA and HITECH regulations and locked into different EHR systems. This creates a silo effect and causes difficulty for interoperation and sharing EHRs. On the other hand, the SHR is open system based on online services, so the data is easily shared over lightweight clients, e.g., a Web browser.

The EHR focuses on individual patients, and it is difficult to connect and aggregate EHRs of many patients unless one has all the access privileges. On the other hand, the SHRs are inherently crowdsourced data due to their base in social

Table 1 Characteristics of EHR and SHR

EHR	SHR
Generated by clinicians or medical experts	Self-reported by patients, public, government
Clinical Data: Diagnoses, prescribed medications, allergies, problems, procedures, chart notes, clinical alert notes, lab results, and images	Experience and Behavior Data: • Health status reports – Experienced symptoms, side effects – Diagnosis reports • Healthcare practice data – Actual medications, treatments • Health-related behaviors/habits – Drinking, smoking, exercises, etc. – Nutritional data
Factual statements	Statements on emotional, psychological attitudes, comments, opinions
Uses medical expert language e.g., Myocardial infarction	Informal everyday language e.g., Heart attack
Comparatively unambiguous e.g., ICD9 code for a disease	Ambiguous or vague e.g., Diabetes (type 1 or 2?) Hepatitis (A or C?)
Closed data – Difficult to share patient data (e.g., due to HIPAA, HITECH regulations) – Often locked in siloed systems	Open data – Membership based sharing – Open sharing – Open system based on Web browsers
Care-oriented	Support-oriented
Individual records	Crowdsourced data

media so they can reveal the aggregated information of the crowd. For instance, the forum entry SHR data in one community group (e.g., cancer patient groups) from many patients may easily reveal the major types of issues and popular treatment options for many patients. The SHRs can provide a unique opportunity to look into health care from the patients' perspectives to identify healthcare-related issues and improve the quality of care. The SHR data from the crowd can facilitate the ability to "connect the dots" among and across many patients and allow gaining public health intelligence and insights, such as detecting disease outbreaks and understanding population-related health trends. The crowdsourced SHRs can be a great asset for public health intelligence. Some examples of potential healthcare benefits of aggregating and mining SHRs include the following:

- determine which health topics are of greatest current concern
- identify a high-risk group of patients
- identify health trends both in the general public and at the individual level
- identify how patients view or feel about particular treatments and practices
- track adverse drug events
- identify the perceived quality of healthcare services, e.g., most desirable outcomes
- create education campaigns and interventions

- offer insights into the relationship between an individual's health and their everyday lifestyles
- reveal patients' attitudes toward health.

These datasets can help to assess and improve healthcare quality, as well as help to modify health-related policies. There are also patient-generated datasets, accessible through social media. Clinicians and healthcare providers may benefit from being aware of national health trends and individual healthcare experiences that are relevant to their current patients. The available open health datasets vary from structured to highly unstructured. Due to this variability, an information seeker has to spend time visiting many, possibly irrelevant, Websites and has to select information from each and integrate it into a coherent mental model.

In this chapter, we discuss an approach to integrating these openly available but widely dispersed health data sources, where health data is created and shared by patients voluntarily, and open knowledge and expertise shared by healthcare providers and professionals. The goal of developing the integrated data sources is to provide answers to information and knowledge needs of end users, to provide insights on public health through diverse analytics on social behaviors, and behavior models learned from the social data to predict trends. The insights are presented to convey an intuitive understanding of the public health trends and alerts for physicians, healthcare staff, health policy workers, and individual patients.

Our approach to integrating diverse open health data sources is through Linked Data principles and Semantic Web technologies. In Sect. 2, we present a brief summary of related works, and in Sects. 3 and 4, we provide the data collection and our approach on how to construct a linked data model which is then used as the basis for developing a set of analytics. In Sect. 5, we present the architecture for our social health data analytics platform and Sect. 6 describes the prototype system and analytics tools. The analytics tools include "Social InfoButtons," which provides awareness of both community and patient health issues, the population health concern trend analyses using machine learning of sentiment classification, and a comorbidity trajectory analysis using tree analysis that may shed light on the population health trends, but also may be useful in predicting a specific patient disease progression. The proposed social health analytics platform provides patients, public health officials, and healthcare specialists with a unified view of health-related information from both official scientific sources and social networks, and provides the capability of exploring the current data along multiple dimensions, such as time and geographical location.

2 Related Works

Integrating data from the Social Web is a challenging task that requires information extraction and data integration. Research works [1–3] extract health information from different sources including the web and social media, sensors, healthcare claims and lab images, and physician notes that provide useful health information. There are still notable differences between professional experts and Web health users. Smith and Wicks [4] found that only 43% of the symptom terms (e.g., PatientsLikeMe) are present in the Unified Medical Language System Metathesaurus (UMLS). Their study reaffirmed the challenges of reconciling the differences between unfettered natural language descriptions and restricted terminologies as well as formalized knowledge sources.

For the data integration, the Semantic Web has been used as a framework for data integration, e.g., Linked Open Data (LOD) [5, 6], to create links between resources distributed in heterogeneous data sources. LOD principles require using URIs to identify resources, RDFs to represent information, and typically use of SPARQL to access the information. Many research works use the Semantic Web for data integration in various fields, e.g., geospatial data integration [7], folksonomies in a social tagging system with an ontology [8] and the fields of solar physics, space physics, and solar terrestrial physics [9]. In health informatics, a semantic integration model of different health data sources is used for annotating social health blogs [10]; a clinical trial knowledge repository is constructed integrating data from clinical trials and from side effect information [11]; and in [12], clinical trial data is integrated with drug data to support end users in finding an appropriate clinical trial for them to participate in.

Even though there are many sentiment analyses of Tweets in general area [13, 14] and in the health domain [15] using data mining and machine learning approach, most of works do not apply the results of the sentiment analysis to measure the degree of public concerns or anxiety toward disease, as an emotional health indicator as we propose.

Data mining and machine learning techniques are used to predict disease risks for individuals or to rank diseases by their risks. For instance, in [16, 17], a condition for one patient is predicted using similar patients, based on 13+ million elderly patients' hospital visit records. In Hassan and Syed [18], collaborative filtering (CF) is used for predicting cardiac death and recurrent myocardial infarction, based on demographics, comorbidity, lab test results, and outcomes from a real-world dataset containing 4557 patients' records. Other studies include the k-means algorithm to cluster patients and applied association rule analysis to predict disease for patients in each cluster [19], the patient risk prediction study in the context of active learning with relative similarities in [20], and the Chronic Disease Recommender System to suggest medical advice and diagnoses to patients [21].

Another set of research attempts to reveal and infer condition progression trajectories. The study in [22] investigated the temporal trajectory patterns of all diseases for the entire country of Denmark, using the Markov Cluster algorithm to identify the five largest clusters of disease trajectories, while a disease progression model is based on a Bipartite Bayesian Network [23] to identify a few comorbidities and infer the progression trajectory and comorbidity onset of individual patients. A number of disease progression models such as path models, oncogenetic tree models, distance-based trees, directed acyclic graph model, etc. are reported in [24]. The progression model for comorbidities we conduct is intended to identify the population-level comorbidity trajectories using large datasets of social media source, using a lightweight tree-based model [25, 26].

3 Multiple Data Sources

The users of public health decision support may include community-based health providers, local, state, and federal government officials as well as the patients. Table 2 summarizes a few typical public health-related questions that these end users may pose to gain public health intelligence for their health decisions.

The content coverage of each individual data source is disparate and not sufficient to address the public health intelligence-related questions shown in Table 2. Table 3 shows the counts of datasets and the content types covered by each individual data source.

PatientsLikeMe, which is a medical, patient-centric, social network, provides patients' personal and medical data and tracks the patients' interactions with their associated conditions, treatments, and symptoms. MedHelp is a platform that hosts

Table 2 SHR-based public health intelligence types

Category	Questions
Statistics	• What are the top conditions with the most patients? • How many patients are suffering from the condition X? • What are the most frequently cited symptoms of the condition X? • What is the percentage distribution of treatment options for the condition X? • Was the public health policy well received (e.g., positive responses) among population groups?
Demographics	• Who are the patients suffering from this condition X? • What is the gender distribution of the patients with X?
Geospatial Analysis	• How are patients with condition X distributed at the state/country level? • What is the average distance to travel for the patients to a treatment facility?
Correlation	• Does gender play a role in choosing treatment options for a condition X? • Is there any difference in treatment options reported in social and official data sources? • Is there any comorbid relationship between two conditions or multiple conditions?
Trends	• What are the changes in the number of cancer type X patients in a community over time by gender? • How did the popular treatments for a condition X change over time, and by location? • How is the disease X spreading in time and by location? • What are the citizens' anxiety level changes over time? • Is our community health improving in terms of morbidity and mortality?

Table 3 Content types in data sources

Data Source	Patient	Condition	Treatment	Symptom	Review	Community	Post	Prevalence
PatientsLikeMe	17,407	1228	5608	2176	n/a	n/a	n/a	n/a
MedHelp	n/a	n/a	n/a	n/a	n/a	365	69,243	n/a
WebMD	n/a	647	180	n/a	86,715	n/a	n/a	n/a
Mayo Clinic	n/a	1116	2496	5426	n/a	n/a	n/a	n/a
CDC	n/a	n/a	n/a	n/a	n/a	n/a	n/a	52

discussion boards (e.g., forums) among patients and health professionals on various aspects of each specific condition or its category. WebMD is an online service providing information about drugs along with users' reviews of each drug, in addition to condition types and typical treatments. The CDC provides statistics of statewide prevalence of diseases. PubMed serves as a repository of comprehensive data on the medical and clinical scientific literature. In many cases, complete publications are accessible. Twitter is a real-time microblogging platform that can be used to monitor disease outbreaks [27] and disease sentiment trends [3], although it is in not healthcare-specific. Among the information provided by Twitter, there are user posts, physical locations, and topics.

In summary, one data source alone may not answer the public health-related questions as shown in Table 2, because each source may cover some content but does not support cross-content queries often needed to gain public health intelligence. In other words, public health intelligence requires, as many applications do, integrated data from disparate data sources, to provide value for different communities and users concerned with questions about public health statistics, trends, correlations, and distributions.

To develop the social health knowledge graph, publicly available data was extracted from *PatientsLikeMe[1]*, *PubMed, WebMD, the* CDC *website*, and the UMLS *Metathesaurus*. The PHP HTML DOM Parser [28] was utilized to extract relevant information from the above websites. The retrieved structured data was stored in a Jena triple store. To extract the relevant PubMed documents about conditions, we searched PubMed using 1228 condition names collected from the PatientsLikeMe list of conditions. For each condition, the available information such as PubMed URL, title, author, and conference/journal of the top 20 matched documents were collected and stored in the Jena triple store. WebMD resources were retrieved in a similar fashion. Furthermore, the CDC BRFSS prevalence data was also collected through scraping, since that data is published in tables, such as the prevalence data of Asthma in 2010 [29].

4   Social Health Knowledge Graph

In order to query any individual social health-related record or to gain public health intelligence, we developed a social health knowledge graph, which serves as integrated knowledge base consisting of health records, extracted from multiple user-generated health contents on their social media data sources and data and expertise (knowledge) from other open health data sources. We use a lightweight ontology that contains the health record-related concepts and relationships, which serves as a semantic schema for integration. Figure 1 shows a snippet of the ontology.

The *Condition, Treatment,* and *Patient* classes are the central concepts in the semantic model. The *Condition* class has the "*isDiagnosedTo*" relationship to the *Patient* class and has the "*exhibit*" relationship to the *Symptom* class, and the

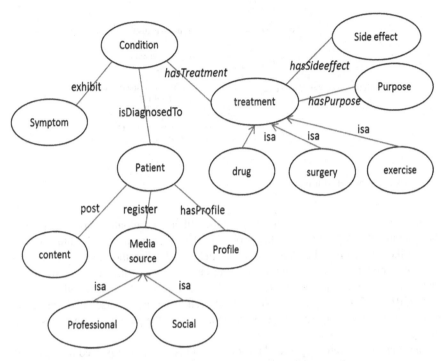

Fig. 1 Social Health Record ontology for semantic integration

"*hasTreatment*" relationship to the *Treatment* class. The *Treatment* class has the "*hasSideEffect*" relationship to the *SideEffect* class and the "*hasPurpose*" relationship to the *Purpose* class. The *Treatment* class also has subclasses indicating different categories of treatments, including *Procedure, Exercise, Drug, Surgery*, etc. The *Drug* class and *Therapy* class also have their own subclasses.

The concepts in the ontology are used to recognize and extract the entities, and the relationships defined in the ontology between concepts help relate the recognized entities.

4.1 Social Health Record Model

Each health record is modeled as a Linked Data assertion represented as a triple *<subject, predicate, object>*, denoting the atomic knowledge unit which states that the "subject" entity is related to the "object" entity by the "predicate" relationship. The subject or object represents a class in ontologies, and a predicate is a property of a class or between classes which states the relationship in existence between two entities. To instantiate the health record model, we extracted the health-related concepts with their URIs and represented them as triples.

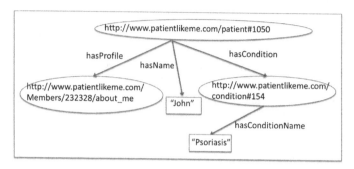

Fig. 2 Example of linked triples

For example, the URI$_1$ at http://www.patientlikeme.com/patient#1050 describes the patient named "John" and his profile is described at the URI$_2$, http://www. patientlikeme.com/members/232328/about_me, and he has the "*Psoriasis*" condition described in URI$_3$ http://www.patientlikeme.com/condition#154. This information is represented as triples <URI$_1$, hasName, John>, <URI$_1$, hasProfile, URI$_2$>, and <URI$_1$ hasCondition URI$_3$>. A group of such triples can be used to describe the patient. The triples corresponding to statements about the patient "John" are shown in Fig. 2.

In order to integrate disparate data sources, entity resolution is used to recognize the terms from different resources that actually represent the same concept. For instance, consider a term for a condition extracted from PatientsLikeMe and another condition retrieved from the CDC website [30]. The PatientsLikeMe condition is referred to "Human immunodeficiency virus", while the CDC refers to it as "HIV". A knowledgeable human can identify these two terms as both referring to the same concept, but for computers, it is harder to capture the underlying identity, especially when two names do not have any literal similarity. For example, "ALS" and "Lou Gehrig's Disease" are two different names but they refer to the same concept.

In general, the problem described above is called the entity consolidation/ resolution or entity disambiguation problem. Rao et al. [31] reviewed the common approaches to entity disambiguation. For entity consolidation in linked open data, Hogan et al. [32] developed a method to use explicit owl:sameAs relations to perform consolidation. In the domain of medical informatics, Hassanzdeh et al. [33] reported on the LinkedCT project, which utilized exact match, string match, and semantic match to discover links between clinical trial entities, such as trials, conditions, interventions, primary outcomes, etc.

As in previous work by Chun and MacKellar [34], the UMLS [35], which contains the Metathesaurus of medical concepts, is used in this research to provide a common vocabulary and semantics for multiple terms that refer to the same concept. Ji et al. [36] developed a term matching algorithm by using the UMLS to recognize identical concepts. CUIs, which are concept unique identifiers for medical concepts in the UMLS, are used by the algorithm to identify the same concept with different terms. To discover the "sameAs" links, we apply two rules: (i) If two

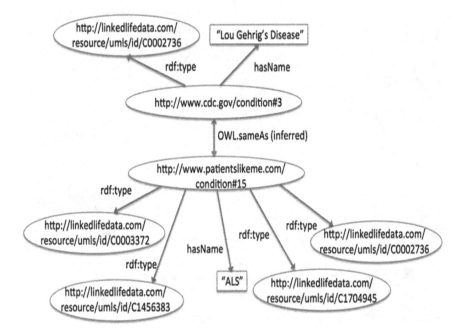

Fig. 3 Entity linking across data sources

conditions in two datasets are of the same name (after necessary stemming and preprocessing), they are regarded as the same concept, and a linkage between the two conditions is discovered; and (ii) When the same CUI is associated with two different condition terms from different datasets, the sameAs link is inferred between the two terms because each concept in the UMLS is uniquely identified by a CUI.

Figure 3 shows that "ALS" from PatientsLikeMe and "Lou Gehrig's Disease" in the UMLS are identified as the same entity, after the sameAs link has been inferred.

5 Architecture of Social Health Analytics Platform

To enable end users like health officials or epidemiologists to draw public health intelligence to better understand the population's health status or to get data-driven insights into the social health behaviors, the *social health analytics platform* is proposed. Figure 4 shows the major components consisting of data extraction, linking, and discovering additional links through inference to construct an integrated connected knowledge graph, and the analytics component where the machine learning component builds the models to automate the data processing to not only summarize, but also to predict sentiments, and diseases that may be correlated with

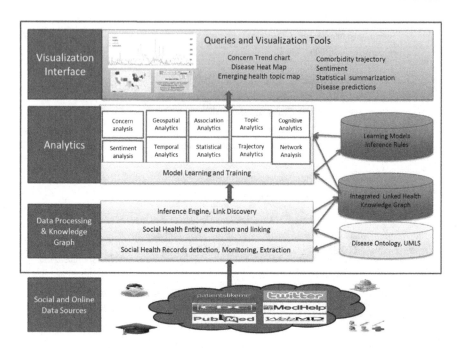

Fig. 4 Social health analytics platform architecture

other diseases. This system is intended to provide answers to various health-related questions as shown in Table 3.

We have implemented a prototype system. The data processing layer at the bottom layer of the architecture is responsible for monitoring the social data sources and extracting and ingesting the data into a staging database. The layer is composed of multiple connectors, one for each type of data source, through APIs or specialized extraction connectors to retrieve data from heterogeneous sources. Among others, we have a Web crawler that uses the PHP HTML DOM Parser to scrape Websites and to retrieve relevant information. Additional connectors can be developed as needed. Data sources currently accessed in our extraction routine include the social network site PatientsLikeMe and Twitter (through APIs), the health forum MedHelp, the government-maintained CDC site, the Mayo Clinic Website, the PubMed Website, and the patient resource portal WebMD. The incoming data, where applicable, goes through the geo-coding processor, where text-based location information is resolved to latitude and longitude coordinates (geo-coding) and, vice versa, coordinates are resolved to names of places (reverse geo-coding) by using third-party services. Geo-coding is required to enable geospatial analytics and to chart data on maps.

Data is then stored in RDF format in the Jena triple store [31] with 612,017 triples representing entities from different sources above mentioned and their relationships. From here, data is linked and augmented via the inference engine component. The latter makes use of supplemental information specified in the UMLS, inference rules repositories, as well as of an entity resolution and a reasoning service. The inference engine is the place where data linkage is performed and additional facts are derived, thus enabling cross-dataset exploration and reasoning about data. Both the inference engine and the triple repository can be accessed via the analytics layer, which is why the analytics are deployed. At the higher level, users interact with the system via visualizations or the system interface, which invokes analytics operations according to the user's input.

6 Social Public Health Analytics

In this section, we provide a few analytical applications using the social health knowledge graph and SHR to illustrate how Social Health Records are used to provide public health intelligence.

6.1 Social InfoButtons

The integrated triple store of social health data can support the basic queries using SPARQL [37]. In addition, to provide answers to the basic queries about public health, the knowledge graph is exploited for knowledge navigation to answer various complex health questions listed in Table 3. It can be used to answer questions such as "What are the top diseases reported by other patients?" or "How many male patients with Asthma are in the state of New Jersey?"

Using these basic capabilities for question answering, we built a Social InfoButtons similar to InfoButtons [38] to provide social health information delivered in a context-aware fashion, e.g., in the clinical patient care context, in the government policy evaluation context, and in the personal information look-up context. Cimino et al. [39, 40] developed InfoButtons to complement the existing Electronic Health Records (EHR) systems and meet the clinicians' information needs in the context of patient care. Cimino et al. [41] described different information needs, their contexts, their resources, and the corresponding applicable methods. In Social InfoButtons, we implemented similar functionalities to provide context-aware information, but the information of Social InfoButtons covers patients' social health information at an aggregated level. This aggregated information includes the percentage of treatments or symptoms for a given disease self-reported by the patients, which can help clinicians to understand the context-specific disease and care patterns or trends from other similar patients at the point of care.

The Social InfoButtons system displays the current disease trends as a list of most common diseases, based on the statistics of the accessed social network sites, as shown in Fig. 5. It also provides disease-specific trends among patients, such as favorite drugs, symptoms, demographics, and geographical distribution of the

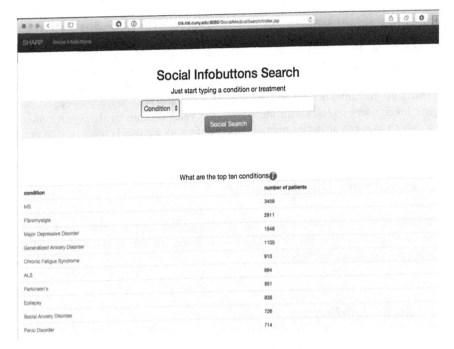

Fig. 5 Social InfoButtons search to provide social health behaviors

patients. The visualization of these social data is juxtaposed with open government data statistics or cutting edge research information from PubMed and WebMD, to allow comparative views.

The social information might be useful for clinicians as it provides them with a new perspective on the current condition/symptoms they are encountering. It is also helpful for patients because when patients are faced with a health concern, they usually want to know how similar patients are coping with the same concern, and how quickly they are recovering.

When a doctor is caring for a veteran who suffers from PTSD (Post-traumatic Stress Disorder), he can practice evidence-based medicine and explore the social trends and experiences of other patients like his patients. As shown in Fig. 6, the Social InfoButtons system can provide answers to typical questions that might be asked by the clinician, represented as information button icons.

This way, the nontechnical person who is not familiar with the SPARQL query language can query the knowledge graph to quickly get the desired answers. For example, the InfoButton icon next to "where is the individual patient?" can provide the doctor with a map (shown in Fig. 7) to indicate the location of all the patients who posted that s/he is suffering from PTSD.

The doctor can look at the total number of patients by region and is able to zoom in on the map for each patient level to view their profile information such as username, social network profile page, gender, age, and location. The treatments

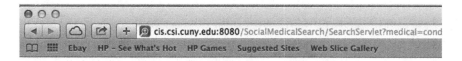

Information of the patients with the condition: PTSD

How many patients? 73

who are these patients? ⓘ

how are the patients distributed in state and country level? ⓘ

where is the indiviual patient? ⓘ

what is the patients' gender distribution? ⓘ

Treatments of the condition: PTSD

Individual Therapy (Psychotherapy)   pubmed   webmed
Evaluated By **95** patients
Side Effects:

Sertraline (Prescription Drug)   pubmed   webmed
Evaluated By **25** patients
Side Effects:
(1) Weight gain 21%;
(2) Dry mouth (xerostomia) 20%;
(3) Loss of sex drive (libido) 18%;
(4) Fatigue 17%;
(5) Insomnia 11%;
(6) Emotional withdrawal 11%;

Citalopram (Prescription Drug)   pubmed   webmed
Evaluated By **22** patients
Side Effects:
(1) Fatigue 25%;
(2) Sex drive (libido) decreased 17%;
(3) Brain fog 15%;
(4) Anxious mood 14%;
(5) Weight gain 13%;
(6) Dizziness 12%;

Fig. 6 PTSD-related Social InfoButtons

used by other similar patients for PTSD and how they reacted to them are also displayed to the doctor to make better informed decisions. For example, if his patient is from a particular location, the doctor can find out common characteristics of all patients in the close-by region, such as any common profile information, notable common symptoms, and treatments reported by other patients. The doctor can make a better recommendation on a treatment regimen that seems more acceptable and more effective to the particular group of patients in the region.

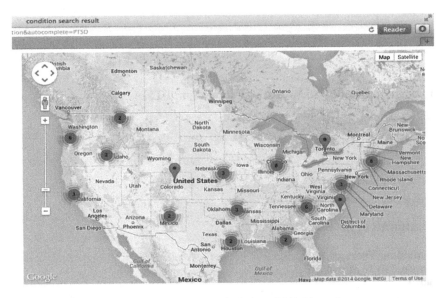

Fig. 7 Map of all patients who reported PTSD in their social health media

For PTSD, the most popular treatment, as shown in Fig. 6, is Individual Therapy, which is a form of Psychotherapy, evaluated by 95 patients, and has no side effect reports. The second most popular treatment, a prescription drug called Sertraline, has side effects such as weight gain (21%) and dry mouth (20%). The doctor can utilize the Social InfoButtons system to retrieve the symptoms and their severity levels. For PTSD, 297 patients reported severe flashbacks, 448 moderate flashbacks, 410 mild flashbacks, and 489 did not report flashbacks. He can compare his patient's symptoms with the other patients and learn that it is most likely his patient's flashback symptoms that may be mild. In summary, the Social InfoButtons system can help doctors to make decisions using knowledge of social trends and experiences of similar patients, using population-level intelligence as a benchmark, and compare it with diagnoses and treatment options for his patient.

A government agency can follow trends and understand whether discrepancies exist between official statistical data and social data. Social InfoButtons can allow officials to identify discrepancies, which may serve as a starting point for further investigations. For instance, there is no universally accepted treatment for Fibromyalgia, a common chronic pain condition. The government official or a researcher can query and browse query results and trigger queries that display analytics of contrasting data from official and social sources for Fibromyalgia. The analytic provides the list of treatments for the condition, ordered by popularity (defined as the number of treatment occurrences in the social space). Starting from this analytic, the knowledge worker can perform a comparison against authoritative sources. For the specific case, the user would discover that a treatment with

Table 4 Discrepancy on treatment types in Social Health Records and authoritative source

Treatment in SI	# of Patients in SI	Appears in Authority
Duloxetine	1058	Yes
Pregabalin	955	Yes
Milnacipran	357	Yes
Gabapentin	346	Yes
Tramadol	201	Yes
Cyclobenzaprine	188	No
Amitriptyline	141	Yes
Hydrocodone–Acetaminophen	128	Yes
Naltrexone	55	No
Massage Therapy	52	No
Meloxicam	50	No
Venlafaxine	46	No
Carisoprodol	43	No

Cyclobenzaprine is reported in social media data but not in official documents, as shown in Table 4.

Similarly, the agency may want to explore the distribution of the population reporting Asthma and how it compares with official data. An interactive map, supplemented with a heat map analysis, allows her to pinpoint the gender distribution by geographical area, and access contrast data via the given charts. Figure 8a, b shows the gender distribution for Asthma in the states of Ohio and Pennsylvania, respectively. From these two figures, it is interesting to note the following: first, there is a substantial difference between data from the official and the social sources; and, second, this difference is consistent across the states, i.e., Ohio and Pennsylvania.

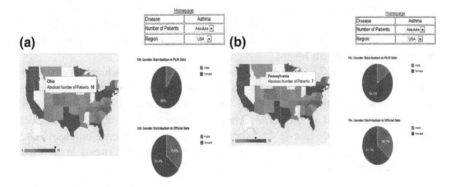

Fig. 8 Asthma distribution heat map and gender breakdown in **a** Ohio and **b** Pennsylvania

In addition, a patient wants to know more about his condition and he is interested in researching the scientific literature, joining social networks, exploring blogs or forums, etc. This can be a challenging task for a nonexpert. The plethora of information channels to consider that pose different levels of terminology issues, and his limited expertise can be prohibitive. Social InfoButtons can help this kind of individual to explore the knowledge, to gain an understanding of crowd level common behaviors or health practices through analytics provided by the system.

6.2 Sentiment Analytics to Monitor Public Health Concerns

We have also developed a sentiment analytics component named ESMOS (Epidemic Sentiment Monitoring System) to monitor the timeline and topic distribution of population-level public health concern [42, 43]. Using Twitter datasets, we developed a sentiment classification model, with unlabeled tweets and the subjective language as well as none-linguistic clues such as emoticons, to distinguish the personal from nonpersonal tweets (e.g., news tweets), and to distinguish positive from negative sentiments among personal tweets. The sentiment analysis results are used to calculate the population-level public concern toward a disease.

The ESMOS displays (1) a concern timeline chart to track the public concern trends on the timeline; (2) a tag cloud for discovering the popular topics within a certain time period with a capability to drill down to the individual tweets; and (3) a public health concern map to show the geographic distribution of particular disease concentrations with different granularities (e.g., state, county, or individual location level).

Figure 9 shows the different visual tools. The public health specialists can utilize the concern timeline chart, as shown in Fig. 9a, to monitor (e.g., identify concern peaks) and compare public concern timeline trends for various diseases. Then the specialists might be interested in what topics people are discussing on social media during the "unusual situations" discovered with the help of the concern timeline chart. To answer this question, they can use the word cloud analytics, as shown in Fig. 9b, to browse the top topics within a certain time period for different diseases and individual tweets. The public health concern heat map in Fig. 9c shows the state-level public concern levels.

This illustrates that Social Health Records, such as tweets, which may be considered as weak signals on their own, can be a source of population-level intelligence to understand the public health issues and attitudes toward a particular disease when analyzed in the large collective datasets. Here, again, each tweet analysis makes use of disease-related knowledge bases (e.g., disease ontology) and subjective language as background knowledge in classifying the tweets in building the classification models.

(a)

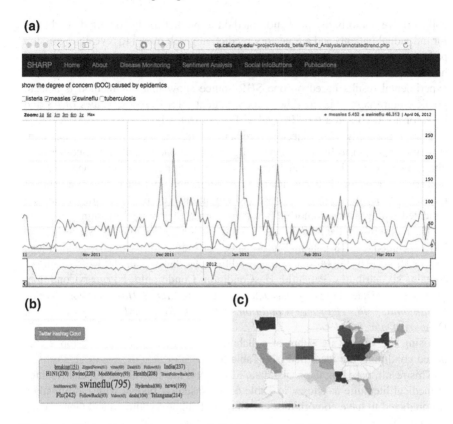

(b)   **(c)**

Fig. 9 **a** Public health concern trend line, **b** Topic trending, **c** Public health concern map

6.3   Comorbidity Prediction and Trajectory Analysis

Managing multiple coexisting conditions of one patient raises important public health issues, especially when conditions are associated with high costs. In the US, 80% of Medicare spending is expended for managing comorbidity of patients. For instance, obese patients often develop type-2 diabetes and hypertension. Thus, predicting potential comorbidity conditions for an individual patient or a group of patients with similar profiles can promote preventive care and reduce costs. In addition, predicting possible comorbidity progression paths using large datasets from the Social Health Records can provide important insights into population health and aid with decisions in public health policies. Discovering the comorbidity relationships is complex and difficult, due to limited access to Electronic Health Records by privacy laws. With the SHRs, great opportunities are provided to study this kind of population-level predictive model building.

In building a prediction model for identifying a potential comorbid condition, or discovering all possible trajectory paths, we take two approaches [25, 26]: a collaborative comorbidity prediction method to predict likely comorbid conditions for individual patients and a trajectory prediction graph model to reveal progression paths of comorbid conditions. Our prediction approaches utilize patient-generated health reports on online social media, i.e., the Social Health Records (SHR). The experimental results based on one SHR source show that our method is able to predict future comorbid conditions for a patient with coverage values of 48 and 75% for a top-20 and a top-100 ranked list, respectively.

For comorbidity risk trajectory prediction, our approach uses a graph construction approach to build a connected graph from one condition to another condition, using edge discovery and linking discovered edges to reveal each potential progression trajectory between any two conditions and infer the confidence value of the future trajectory, given any observed condition. The predicted trajectories are validated with existing comorbidity relations from the medical literature.

The dataset from the patients' self-posted data on the PatientsLikeMe website in 2012 included 17,418 patients' information, including id, username, gender, age, and location, and 35,606 diagnosed conditions for these patients. Each diagnosis contains six attributes: PatientId, HasCondition, ConditionId, IsPrimaryCondition, FirstSymptomDate, and DiagnosisDate, for example, "*ID: 8, HasCondition: Stroke, ConditionId: 48, IsPrimaryCondition: 0, FirstSymptomDate: May 1998, DiagnosisDate: Sep 1998*".

Using the variant algorithm of collaborative filtering approach, the top 2 predicted conditions are identified (see Table 5).

This result, based on the social data, has a good match with the official findings in medical literature as shown in Table 6. For instance, people with Fibromyalgia are predicted to have comorbidities of Chronic Fatigue Syndrome and Generalized Anxiety Disorder.

However, the medical literature results or the collaborative prediction model do not show the possible trajectory to show the progress from one condition to another, other than stating that these conditions likely co-occur.

The trajectory analyses using the SHRs have shown more promising transitional steps of the comorbidity direction. The following visual analysis using our approach in Fig. 10 shows the trajectory of the potential comorbidity progression for public health insights, using collective intelligence garnered from a large set of SHR records from many people.

Figure 10 shows the progression trajectory starting with "Major Depressive Disorder" (MDD). The numbers in parentheses on each node indicate the numbers

Table 5 Example of predicted comorbidity conditions associated with diagnosed conditions

Id	Diagnosed Conditions	Top 2 Predicted Conditions
296	Migraine, **Fibromyalgia**	**Chronic Fatigue Syndrome, Generalized Anxiety Disorder**
42	Eating Disorder, Phobic disorder	Social Anxiety Disorder, PTSD
50	HIV, Seborrheic Dermatitis	Bipolar Disorder, Lactose Intolerance

Table 6 Comorbidities from medical literature

Condition Category	Comorbidity
Major Depressive Disorder (MDD)	Dysthymia, Panic Disorder, Agoraphobia, Social Anxiety, Obsessive–Compulsive Disorder, Generalized Anxiety Disorder, and Post-traumatic Stress Disorder, Alcohol Dependence, Psychotic Disorder, Antisocial personality, Eating Disorders, Borderline Personality Disorder
Irritable Bowel Syndrome (IBS)	Major Depression, **Anxiety**, Somatoform Disorders, **Fibromyalgia**, **Chronic Fatigue Syndrome**, Gastroesophageal Reflux Disease, Restless Legs Syndrome

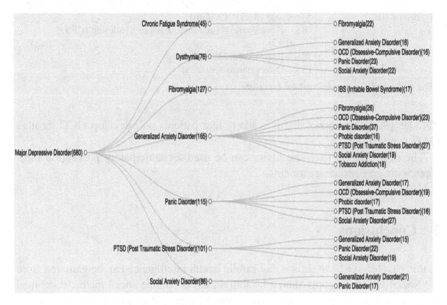

Fig. 10 The comorbidity progression trajectory model starting from "Major Depressive Disorder"

of patients following the trajectory from the root to the current node, e.g., there are 17 patients with the trajectory (MDD→Fibromyalgia→IBS). In Fig. 3, the most frequent length-2 trajectories are (MDD→GAD) (165 patients) followed by (MDD→Fibromyalgia) (127 patients). The most frequent length-3 trajectory is (MDD→GAD→PD) (PD = Panic Disorder). The confidence value of (MDD→GAD→Panic Disorder), given the observed condition MDD, is $37/680 = 5.4\%$. The other length-3 trajectories between MDD and PD are (MDD→Dysthymia→PD) (3.4%), followed by (MDD→PTSD→PD) (3.2%) and (MDD→Social Anxiety Disorder→PD) (2.5%).

This comorbidity progression trajectory analysis results from our study as shown in Table 7 contrasting with those in Table 6, where the comorbid conditions are just listed without showing the progression. For instance, the trajectory MDD→Generalized Anxiety Disorder (GAD)*→Obsessive–Compulsive Disorder

Table 7 Trajectory analysis results for comorbidity prediction (comorbidity index in percentage/confidence value in percentage/support)

Condition	Comorbidity
Major Depressive Disorder (MDD)	MDD→Post-traumatic Stress Disorder (PTSD)*→Panic Disorder*→Social Anxiety Disorder* (0.25/1.3/9) MDD→PD*→SAD*→Phobic Disorder (0.23/1.1/8) MDD→Generalized Anxiety Disorder (GAD)*→Obsessive–Compulsive Disorder (OCD)* (0.7/3/23) MDD→PD*→OCD* (0.7/2/19) MDD→Bipolar II (1.7/4/21) MDD→Borderline Personality Disorder* (1.2/3/21)
Irritable Bowel Syndrome (IBS)	IBS→Gastroesophageal Reflux Disease (GERD)*→Restless Legs Syndrome (RLS)* (0.9/3/6) IBS→Fibromyalgia*→Chronic Fatigue Syndrome (CFS)* (0.3/9/17) IBS→RLS* (6/12/23) IBS→Osteoarthritis (3/10/18)

*The comorbidity exists in medical literature

(OCD)* (0.7/3/23) shows that it is likely that patients will develop OCD through GAD from MDD.

The new insights from the SHRs can be used for anticipatory prevention measures with appropriate treatments.

7 Conclusions

In this chapter, we have shown that public health intelligence can be gathered from the Social Health Records shared by individuals on online social media, combined with the authoritative data shared by medical experts. We have presented a Social Health Analytics Platform for enabling the use of semantics in the analysis of Social Health Records to gain population-level health intelligence. The proposed Social Health Records Analytics Platform enables flexible collection of data from a variety of sources. Collected data is reconciled in a unified data model focusing on medical conditions and treatments and linked to create a knowledge base that enables cross-dataset exploration and analysis. Furthermore, the knowledge base can be extended by defining inference rules and using automatic reasoning.

We have illustrated the Social Health Analytics cases for population health, including the Social InfoButtons application to provide on-demand social health intelligence according to the information needs in different situations, sentiment analysis of Social Health Records to measure the population level of concern for health issues, and visual and trending analytics to provide situation awareness of disease evolution. We further discussed the comorbid progression analytics to predict the likely conditions to develop and the likely paths from one condition to another through time. The content of each individual Social Health Record

(SHR) may not provide many insights, but we showed that collectively the SHRs can bring great value for population health intelligence and understanding.

Many challenges still exist with using SHRs, because the data governance issues such as who owns the SHRs and who decides to share them need to be further addressed. So far, the use the SHRs has been relatively free of any governmental regulations and is subject to the data policies of online social media providers. However, there is concern that the existing privacy issues may prevent the effective utilization of SHRs for analytics in the future.

Acknowledgements The research work reported in this paper was partially funded by PSC-CUNY Research Foundation under the award numbers #64266 and #65232. The main research was carried out as part of the dissertation work by X. Ji at NJIT. The dataset was collected in the year 2012 when it is freely available. The data was processed right after.

References

1. Raghupathi, W., Raghupathi, V.: Big data analytics in healthcare: promise and potential. Health Inf. Sci. Syst. **2**, 1–10 (2014)
2. Househ, M., Borycki, E., Kushniruk, A.: Empowering patients through social media: the benefits and challenges. Health Inf. J. **20**, 50–58 (2014)
3. Ji X, Chun, S.A., Geller, J.: Monitoring public health concerns using Twitter sentiment classifications. In: Proceedings of IEEE International Conference on Healthcare Informatics, pp. 335–344. Philadelphia, PA (2013)
4. Smith, C.A., Wicks, P.J.: PatientsLikeMe: consumer health vocabulary as a folksonomy. In: Proceedings of American Medical Informatics Association Annual Symposium, pp. 682–686. Washington D.C. (2008)
5. Bizer, C.: Evolving the web into a global data space. In: Fernandes, A.A., Gray, A.G., Belhajjame, K. (eds.) Proceedings of 28th British National Conference on Databases, p. 1. Springer, Manchester, UK (2011)
6. Bizer, C., Heath, T., Berners-Lee, T.: Linked data—the story so far. Int. J. Semant. Web Inf. Syst. **5**, 1–22 (2009)
7. Harth, A., Gil, Y.: Geospatial data integration with linked data and provenance tracking. In: W3C/OGC Linking Geospatial Data Workshop, pp. 1–5 (2014)
8. Specia, L., Motta, E.: Integrating folksonomies with the semantic web. In: Proceedings of the 4th European Conference on The Semantic Web: Research and Applications, pp. 624–639. Springer, Innsbruck, Austria (2007)
9. Fox, P., McGuinness, D.L., Cinquini, L., et al.: Ontology-supported scientific data frameworks: the virtual solar-terrestrial observatory experience. Comput. Geosci. **35**, 724–738 (2009)
10. Chun, S.A., MacKellar, B.: Social health data integration using semantic Web. In: Proceedings of the 27th Annual ACM Symposium on Applied Computing, pp. 392–397 (2012)
11. MacKellar, B., Schweikert, C., Chun, S.A.: Patient-centered clinical trials decision support using linked open data. Int. J. Softw. Sci. Comput. Intell. **6**, 31–48 (2014)
12. Tofferi, J.K., Jackson, J.L., O'Malley, P.G.: Treatment of fibromyalgia with cyclobenzaprine: a meta-analysis. Arthritis Rheum. **51**, 9–13 (2004)
13. Pang, B., Lee, L.: Opinion mining and sentiment analysis. Found. Trends Inf. Retrieval **2**(1–2), 1–135 (2008)

14. Zhuang, L., Jing, F., Zhu, X.-Y.: Movie review mining and summarization. In: Proceedings of the 15th ACM International Conference on Information and Knowledge Management, pp. 43–50. Arlington, VAS (2006)
15. Chew, C., Eysenbach, G.: Pandemics in the age of Twitter: content analysis of Tweets during the 2009 H1N1 outbreak. PLoS ONE **5**(11), e14118 (2010)
16. Chawla, N.V., Davis, D.A.: Bringing big data to personalized healthcare: a patient-centered framework. J. Gen. Intern. Med. **28**, 660–665 (2013)
17. Davis, D.A., Chawla, N.V., Christakis, N.A., Barabasi, A.L.: Time to CARE: a collaborative engine for practical disease prediction. Data Min. Knowl. Disc. **20**, 388–415 (2010)
18. S. Hassan and Z. Syed, "From netflix to heart attacks: collaborative filtering in medical datasets," in *Proceedings of the 1st ACM International Health Informatics Symposium*, Arlington, Virginia, USA, 2010, pp. 128–134
19. Folino, F., Pizzuti, C.: A comorbidity-based recommendation engine for disease prediction. In: Proceedings of the IEEE 23rd International Symposium on Computer-Based Medical Systems, pp. 6–12. Bentley, Australia (2010)
20. Qian, B., Wang, X., Cao, N., Li, H., Jiang, Y.-G.: A relative similarity based method for interactive patient risk prediction. Data Min. Knowl. Disc. **29**, 1070–1093 (2015)
21. Hussein, A.S., Omar, W.M., Li, X., Hatem, M.A.: Smart collaboration framework for managing chronic disease using recommender system. Health Syst. **3**, 12–17 (2014)
22. Jensen, A.B., Moseley, P.L., Oprea, T.I., Ellesøe, S.G., Eriksson, R., Schmock, H., et al.: Temporal disease trajectories condensed from population-wide registry data covering 6.2 million patients. Nat. Commun. **5** (2014)
23. Wang, X., Sontag, D., Wang, F.: Unsupervised learning of disease progression models. In: Proceedings of the 20th ACM SIGKDD International Conference on Knowledge Discovery and Data Mining, pp. 85–94. New York, NY (2014)
24. Hainke, K., Rahnenführer, J., Fried, R.: Disease progression models: a review and comparison. Dortmund University, Technical Report (2011)
25. Ji, X., Chun, S.A., Geller, J., Oria, V.: Collaborative and trajectory prediction models of medical conditions by mining patients' social data. In: Proceedings of 2015 IEEE International Conference on Bioinformatics and Biomedicine (BIBM), pp. 695–700. Washington D.C. (2015)
26. Ji, X., Chun, S., Geller, J.: Predicting comorbid conditions and trajectories using social health records. IEEE Trans. Nanobiosci. **15**(4):371–379 (2016)
27. Ji, X., Chun, S.A., Geller, J.: Epidemic outbreak and spread detection system based on twitter data. In: Proceedings of the First International Conference on Health Information Science, pp. 152–163. Beijing, China (2012)
28. PHP Simple HTML DOM Parser. http://simplehtmldom.sourceforge.net. Accessed 14 Apr 2014
29. CDC Prevalence Data of Asthma in 2010. http://www.cdc.gov/asthma/brfss/2010/brfssdata.htm. Accessed 14 Apr 2014
30. Behavioral Risk Factor Surveillance System. http://www.cdc.gov/brfss/. Accessed 14 Apr 2014
31. Rao, D., McNamee, P., Dredze, M.: Entity linking: finding extracted entities in a knowledge base. In: Poibeau, T., Saggion, H., Piskorski, J., Yangarber, R. (eds.) Multi-source, Multilingual Information Extraction and Summarization. Theory and Applications of Natural Language Processing, pp. 93–115. Springer, Berlin (2013)
32. Hogan, A., Zimmermann, A., Umbrich, J., Polleres, A., Decker, S.: Scalable and distributed methods for entity matching, consolidation and disambiguation over linked data corpora. Web Semant. **10**, 76–110 (2012). doi:10.1016/j.websem.2011.11.002
33. Hassanzadeh, O., Kementsietsidis, A., Lim, L., Miller, R.J., Wang, M.: LinkedCT: a linked data space for clinical trials. CoRR **abs/0908.0567** (2009)
34. Chun, S.A., MacKellar, B.: Social health data integration using semantic Web. In: Proceedings of the 27th Annual ACM Symposium on Applied Computing, pp. 392–397. Trento, Italy (2012)

35. Bodenreider, O.: The Unified Medical Language System (UMLS): integrating biomedical terminology. Nucleic Acids Res. **32**(Database issue), D267–270 (2004). doi:10.1093/nar/gkh061
36. Ji, X., Chun, S.A., Geller, J.: Social InfoButtons: integrating open health data with social data using semantic technology. In: Proceedings of the Fifth Workshop on Semantic Web Information Management, New York (2013)
37. SPARQL Query Language for RDF. http://www.w3.org/TR/rdf-sparql-query/. Accessed 14 Apr 2014
38. Collins, S.A., Currie, L.M., Bakken, S., Cimino, J.J.: Information needs, Infobutton Manager use, and satisfaction by clinician type: a case study. (1067–5027 (Print)) (2009)
39. Cimino, J.J., Elhanan, G., Zeng, Q.: Supporting infobuttons with terminological knowledge. In: Proceedings of AMIA Annual Fall Symposium, pp. 528–532. AMIA, Bethesda, MD (1997)
40. Cimino, J.J.: Use, usability, usefulness, and impact of an infobutton manager. In: Proceedings of American Medical Informatics Association Annual Symposium, pp. 151–155. AMIA, Bethesda, MD (2006)
41. Cimino, J.J., Li, J., Allen, M., Currie, L.M., Graham, M., Janetzki, V., Lee, N.J., Bakken, S., Patel, V.L.: Practical considerations for exploiting the World Wide Web to create infobuttons. Medinfo **11**, 277–281 (2004)
42. Ji, X., Chun, S.A., Wei, Z., Geller, J.: Twitter sentiment classification for measuring public health concerns. Soc. Netw. Anal. Min. **5**, 1–25 (2015)
43. Ji, X., Chun, S., Geller, J.: Knowledge-based tweet classification for disease sentiment monitoring. In: Pedrycz, W., Chen S.-M. (eds.) Sentiment Analysis and Ontology Engineering: An Environment of Computational Intelligence, pp. 425–454. Springer (2016)

Using Dynamic Bayesian Networks for Incorporating Nontraditional Data Sources in Public Health Surveillance

Masoumeh Izadi, Katia Charland and David L. Buckeridge

Abstract The estimation of disease prevalence based on public health surveillance data requires the accurate identification of cases from limited information (e.g., diagnostic codes). These data sources typically consist of routinely collected records of population healthcare utilization, such as administrative and clinical data, that specifies diagnostic codes or terms for each encounter. These data sources include, for example, emergency department visits, pharmaceutical (drug) dispensations, and laboratory test orders. The case definitions depend on the data source and are typically based on the presence of diagnostic codes or key words in a prespecified time frame. Each data source will result in a certain degree of misclassification bias when estimating prevalence. Inaccuracies can occur at each stage from the time the disease process is initiated to the stage at which diagnostic codes are entered into the database. Indeed, when relying on these data sources, asymptomatic cases will be missed, as well as those not seeking health care. Even patients that seek care may be inaccurately diagnosed or the diagnostic code that is entered in the system may not represent the diagnosis or may not be a code or key word used in the definition. In addition to misclassification bias, these data sources are not usually available in a timely manner. Timeliness is an important factor for prevalence estimation in certain contexts such as the prevalence of infectious diseases during an epidemic. For instance, in an influenza pandemic, such estimates must be obtained within days. In recent years, several nonclinical and nontraditional data sources have been introduced to public health surveillance with the potential to provide more timely signals of changing prevalence trends. Ideally, combining the

M. Izadi (✉) · K. Charland
Clinical and Health Informatics Research Group, McGill University,
Montreal, QC, Canada
e-mail: mtabae@cs.mcgill.ca

K. Charland
e-mail: katia.charland@mcgill.ca

D.L. Buckeridge
Department of Epidemiology & Biostatistics and Occupational Health,
McGill University, Montreal, QC, Canada
e-mail: david.buckeridge@mcgill.ca

© Springer International Publishing AG 2017
A. Shaban-Nejad et al. (eds.), *Public Health Intelligence and the Internet*,
Lecture Notes in Social Networks, https://doi.org/10.1007/978-3-319-68604-2_3

new and traditional data sources, there is greater potential to overcome bias and provide more timely signals. However, building a construct capable of incorporating data from these various sources in a coherent manner is not trivial. In this research, we consider the case of the 2009–2010 H1N1 pandemic as the context of interest and we use media reports of deaths from H1N1 on the web as a nontraditional data source. We propose to use dynamic Bayesian networks from the class of probabilistic graphical models in order to combine this new data source with traditional ones through exploration of the possible probabilistic relationships between these data streams. This is an initial step toward building a framework that can potentially support aggregation of heterogeneous data for a real-time estimation of disease prevalence. Our preliminary results show that the proposed model can be used in accurate prediction of short-term future counts of the data sources. This is particularly useful in timely prediction of epidemic changes over a defined population.

Keywords Public health · Surveillance systems · Probabilistic models · Nontraditional data sources · Dynamic Bayesian networks

1   Introduction

Infectious disease outbreaks result in high human and financial costs. Respiratory and gastrointestinal infectious diseases, in particular, are among the most prevalent types of infections encountered in routine public health practice. The rapid emergence of the novel pandemic (H1N1) 2009 influenza virus in the spring of 2009 gave rise to a pandemic that resulted in more than 18,000 deaths [1]. Due to the continued threat of influenza and recognizing the importance of methodological advances to provide timely and accurate estimates of disease burden, building models that can synthesize the information from diverse data sources is crucial. Several streams of data such as the volume of visits to emergency departments, sales of over-the-counter drugs, call volume to health information lines, and the number of admissions to hospitals are routinely used for monitoring outbreaks. In addition, advances in public health surveillance research have included the identification and validation of novel data sources for monitoring infectious diseases. Despite the wealth of information from these diverse data streams that may be synthesized to form a comprehensive estimate of disease prevalence, the majority of surveillance systems responsible for monitoring changes in disease burden from these data assess disease prevalence from each data source separately or combine estimates in an ad hoc fashion.

Synthesizing the information from the data sources can increase statistical power and alleviate biases due to confounding and misclassification, in general. Combining heterogeneous data sources has become the focus of extensive theoretical work and numerous applications. Multiple kernels learning [2], N-dimensional order statistics (NDOS) method [3], and Bayesian propensity score have been used for combining data sources. Bayesian network framework also has been used recently for combining heterogeneous data for accurate prediction of protein function, in bioinformatics research. However, combining temporal data introduces another layer of complexity to integrating data sources. Building an architecture to aggregate such data from different sources in a way that can be easily used for reasoning and prediction is not always easy. Moreover, the desired architecture must be scalable, easily updated, extensible, and more importantly, accurate for prediction of the associated time series.

Classical approaches to time series prediction include linear models such as ARIMA (autoregressive integrated moving average) [4, 5], ARMAX (Autoregressive Moving Average Exogenous Variables Model), and nonlinear models such as neural networks and decision trees. Problems with these approaches include the fact that it is difficult to incorporate prior knowledge and multidimensional sources into the same model. We address this problem using probabilistic graphical models which can be used as tools for fusion of data sources while they allow domain knowledge integration as well [6].

Probabilistic graphical models are represented by a graph with nodes and links, where nodes represent variables of interest and links indicate probabilistic relationships among nodes. These models show great potential for data mining, knowledge discovery, and data analysis. The main advantage of these models is that their underlying graph structure, which conveys the probabilistic relationships for any number of variables, is learned from the data, or can be selected by the experts, or both. Bayesian networks (BNs) and hidden Markov models (HMMs) are among the most popular forms of these models. Both models provide promising methodologies for encoding relations among a large number of random variables based on the conditional independence property and they are able to represent real-world problems with a high degree of complexity. A generalization of these two models is known as dynamic Bayesian networks (DBNs). DBNs generalize Bayesian networks to model temporal relations and generalize HMMs to model interdependencies between observations.

Our objective in this research is to create a DBN as a unified model to combine and mine different data streams relevant to the influenza pandemic. After these relationships between the data streams are learned and the model is built, it can be used for inference and predictions. Another important issue we would like to address is the problem of timeliness. It is especially important in the case of epidemics to forecast prevalence with enough lead time to allow for preparation. In this paper, we show that there is no need to wait for a week or more in order to forecast influenza burden.

To further elucidate upon the utility of DBNs in the context of synthesizing the information from diverse data sources to estimate infectious disease burden, we describe a case study of influenza surveillance in which DBNs were used to provide timely and accurate estimates of influenza burden. Our investigations are based on available administrative data sources that provide information related to the incidence rate of H1N1 over the pandemic and non-pandemic periods. For illustration purposes, in our case study, we focus on the data from the island of Montreal, in the province of Quebec in Canada. However, our approach is easily extendable to other geographical locations and other surveillance situations. The steps in the reasoning and prediction by these models will be illustrated through the H1N1 case study in this paper.

2   Traditional and Nontraditional Data Sources for Influenza Surveillance

Advanced surveillance systems, including the US Influenza Surveillance System and the Public Health Agency of Canada's FluWatch, collect five types of surveillance data: virologic, outpatient visits for influenza-like illnesses, influenza-associated hospitalizations, influenza- and pneumonia-related deaths, and geographic spread of influenza. Also, reports submitted to public health departments on a regular basis, from collaborating laboratories, on the total number of specimens testing positive for influenza, are another routinely collected source of data for influenza surveillance.

There are other data streams that have the potential for integration into surveillance systems including over-the-counter drug sales, 911 calls, ambulatory dispatch, calls to medical helplines, and school and work absenteeism records. The importance of incorporating such sources is noted through the body of literature on assessing the value of such data [7, 8]. Ongoing investigations are performed to explore the most effective means of data fusion and the most informative and timely data streams [9].

Internet-based sources of data have gained a lot of attention from surveillance researchers and practitioners, over the last few years. This is due to the fact that such data sources have demonstrated correlations with the actual clinical data in the case of influenza [9]. Queries to online search engines have been used to track influenza-like illness in a population. Online news sites, social networks, blogs, and discussion forums have increased in number, volume, and coverage, and show potential as useful data sources for disease surveillance [4, 7, 10]. Evidence exists to support the idea that Internet-based data sources may improve the timeliness of detection. Major outbreaks investigated by the World Health Organization (WHO) are first identified through these Internet-based sources [8, 11]. However, Internet-based data sources are not well organized. Tools need to be developed in order to parse, annotate, and assimilate a broad range and a large number of pages as appearing online, constantly. HealthMap [10] is one of these developed tools that assist event-based monitoring of infectious diseases for surveillance purposes by leveraging Internet news and other electronic media. We used HealthMap to extract nontraditional data for the case study of H1N1 surveillance studied in this paper.

3 Dynamic Bayesian Networks

Bayesian networks (BNs) provide a compact representation for expressing joint probability distributions and for probabilistic inference [12–14]. They have gained increasing popularity in the biological sciences [9]. The representation and use of probability theory make BNs suitable for combining domain knowledge and observational data, expressing causal relationships, and learning from incomplete datasets.

A Bayesian network is represented by a Directed Acyclic Graph (DAG). The DAG contains nodes for each random variable considered in a problem and links between any two statistically correlated nodes. The node originating the directed link is a parent and the terminating node a child. Therefore, the DAG explicitly represents conditional independence relationships among the random variables. The existence of a link between two nodes represents the conditional dependence between the corresponding variables. Each node contains a conditional probability table (CPT) that describes the relationship between the node and its parents. If the topology of the DAG (i.e., the structure of the network) is unknown, then the independence relations among the random variables are unknown and an appropriate structure must be elicited from the data or from domain knowledge.

Automatically learning the structure of a Bayesian network DAG from data is a well-researched but computationally difficult problem [15, 16]. Conceptually, a function is used to score a network with respect to the training data, and a search method is used to look for the network structure with the best score. Different scoring metrics and search methods have been proposed in the literature. The scoring functions used to select models are based on the likelihood function of a model, given the data or the logarithm of this function. Since the associated search space is exponentially large, local search-based approaches, which iteratively consider local changes (adding, deleting, and reversing an edge) to the network structure, are usually used to find the best network topology. This type of search is very useful when dealing with large datasets because of its computational efficiency. One of the most popular search strategies due to its simplicity and good performance in this context is the greedy hill-climbing search [17] which starts from an empty graph and gradually improves it by applying the highest scoring single edge addition or removal available.

Once the DAG is learned, the parameters of the model (CPTs) need to be specified or directly learned from data. CPTs identify the probabilities of the child being in any specific values given the values of its parents. Parameter learning in Bayesian networks mainly considers maximum likelihood estimation of the model given the data and it is performed through an expectation maximization process. See [18, 19] for parameter learning methods in Bayesian networks.

A DBN consists of a finite number of BNs called slices, where each slice corresponds to a particular time instant. BNs corresponding to successive instants are connected through arcs that represent how the state of a random variable changes over time. A DBN is generally assumed to satisfy Markov (or k-Markov) property. This means that temporally, each node only depends on the nodes one (or up to k) time step earlier. It is generally assumed that the dependencies between the nodes on one slice of a DBN, which present a BN, do not change over time. Therefore, a DBN can be described by at most a k-slice network (for a k-order Markov domain). The advantage of DBNs is being able to represent uncertainties, dependencies, and dynamics exhibited in different time series.

DBNs have been applied in a variety of applications from activity recognition and monitoring to medical diagnosis and fault or defect detection. DBNs have also been used for inferring genetic regulatory interactions from microarray data. To our knowledge, this is the first time that this framework is used for mining in epidemiological data. Ideally, we should be able to learn and discover the probabilistic relationships between data streams through structure learning in DBNs. However, when the system consists of many data streams and in particular when it is partially observed, structure learning in DBNs becomes computationally intensive. This is due to the fact that the space of possible models is so huge that it will be necessary to use strong prior domain knowledge to make the task tractable. To design a DBN structure that adequately reflects relationships between evidence from different data types for the purpose of ensemble analysis, we used statistical techniques explained in Sect. 5.

4 Data

Through collaborations with the department of public health in Montreal, we had access to five different surveillance data sources. These data sources include daily counts of emergency department visits, daily counts of calls to health information lines (Info-Sante), weekly counts of H1N1 vaccination, weekly counts of confirmed cases of H1N1 through lab tests, and weekly counts of admission to the hospitals. Several quantitative relationships between some of these data sources are also known as domain knowledge.

The data sources available to us come with different resolutions in time and have a varying time delay. Therefore, for the purpose of consistency, in preliminary analyses, we only considered the data sources that were reported on a daily basis. This includes daily time series of emergency department (ED) visits and calls to health lines (Info-Sante). Quebec's Info-Sante (IS) is available to all residents of the province. Users are encouraged to call with any general health questions and confidential advice is given regarding their health concerns. The system is available 24 h per day. Healthcare recommendations are made by trained and experienced registered nurses. We conducted data extraction for Influenza-like illness (ILI) complaints in IS calls for a period of time in which the H1N1 pandemic period was a subset. Anonymized data was obtained from this data source. We aggregated ILI calls by age group, sex, and day of the call. Similar to the ED data, the IS data can be used to assess temporal patterns in influenza burden.

We also utilized an Internet-based data as a nonconventional source for H1N1 infection monitoring. Media reports of deaths from pandemic H1N1 were considered important because of their pronounced effect on the utilization of health services, thus media reports were filtered for content. We used HealthMap as a web-based tool for data collection on localized instances of H1N1. We extracted the media data from the HealthMap [10] on a daily basis.

5 Methods

We applied and evaluated DBNs in the context of data integration from different sources which partially indicate the patterns of Influenza H1N1 infection. There are natural relationships between infection rate or influenza-like-illness incidence and other data sources to which we have access, such as vaccination data. Influenza infections are thought to make up approximately one-third of influenza-like-illness infections so vaccination against influenza would likely reduce the volume of healthcare visits for ILI. While very useful, these diverse pieces of information alone are not sufficient to establish a comprehensive model. DBNs are capable of incorporating such domain knowledge in their structure while they build on the knowledge discovered by the data.

Although conventionally DBNs are based on first-order Markov processes (i.e., they can be implemented by one-step temporal relationships between two static BNs), we were advised that the data sources we have considered in this work may potentially indicate more than one-step lag between the time series. Therefore, embedding of this particular information into a DBN formulation requires a k-order Markov process for representing a k-layer Bayesian network, where k indicates the maximum lag between the time series.

Our approach to uncovering the relationships between the time series is to first use statistical techniques to assess the extent of lead–lag relationships among the data sources. We then combined that with domain knowledge, and then use this information to construct the required DBN.

We used a statistical technique called Wavelet Coherency Analysis (WCA) [20, 21] to estimate the extent of any lead–lag relationships between the data streams. Wavelet coherency analysis is a useful technique for analyzing periodicities in longitudinal data [22–24]. Though it has many applications, WCA is especially useful in highlighting the time and frequency intervals in which two time series show substantial synchrony.

In the case of our time series, wavelet coherency is useful at finding synchrony in the anomalies of the series. The series are nonstationary and thus show large-scale trends. We assess synchrony in the series after removing these large-scale trends. Coherence is defined as the cross-spectrum normalized to an individual power spectrum. It is a number between 0 and 1, and results in a measurement of the cross-correlation between two time series and a frequency function. Wavelet-squared coherency is a measure of the intensity of the covariance of the two series in time–frequency space [25]. It is used to identify frequency bands within which two time series are covarying. The WCA can identify pairs of series that display temporal relationships that warrant further exploration in the Bayesian network setting. This is done via the computation of time–frequency maps of the time-variant coherence [23].

The development of DBNs is based on the data presented in the paper. In all our investigations, we enforced the presence of the arcs in the DBN network structure based on the suggested settings by WCA, or BN structure learning. We learned DBN models from the data in a variety of settings and compared them with respect to their performance in predicting the future observable data streams. The main purpose of this phase of the research is to understand how well DBNs can represent the whole picture, a unified view of the information in the observed data sources. We also explored different settings to empirically show how many observations are required and what which observations are most useful.

In performing the BN structure learning, we followed a similar strategy to that suggested by Sebastiani et al. [9]. For each data source, we selected the variables observed at t, t+1... t+10 days and performed hill-climbing searches to identify the network with the best score.

6   Results

Figure 1 shows the total daily counts of H1N1 media reports about Montreal during the period of April 28, 2009, to December 16, 2009, in the top graph.

The second graph depicts the total daily calls to IS, and the third graph shows the total daily counts of emergency department visits during the same period. The arrow points to the time when a 13-year-old boy (hockey player) in Ontario died on October 26. There were reports of his funeral at around November 4 (t = 203 on the time axis). This precedes, by 1 day, the sharp spike in IS calls.

The extent of the temporal relationship between IS and ED data series was estimated using WCA in Fig. 2. Our results in Fig. 2 show about 2–4-day lead (or lag). The US Influenza Surveillance System identified two distinct waves of pandemic influenza H1N1 activity, the first peaking in June 2009, followed by a second peak in October 2009. All our influenza surveillance data showed levels of influenza activity above that typically seen during late summer and early fall. There is a phase change at around Nov 2, in the second wave. We are able to see a predictable relationship during seasonal influenza (with IS leading ED by approximately 4 days), but during the pandemic (and especially the second wave) the relationship was less predictable. We speculated that it is possibly due to media influence.

The first set of experiments involved learning DBNs of different complexities. We used a BN structure learning search over the space of all possible graphs to find the best graph, and we discovered 2-day lag for ED during the seasonal and pandemic flu 2009 (see Fig. 3). However, for an extended period of time (May 1, 2008, to December 30, 2009), which includes non-pandemic, seasonal, and pandemic flu,

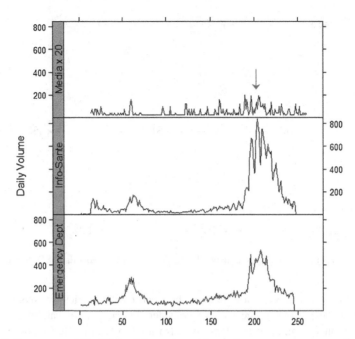

Fig. 1 Daily counts of HealthMap Montreal-specific media reports, emergency department (ED) visits and calls to the health information line, IS, in Montreal between April 28, 2009, and December 16, 2009

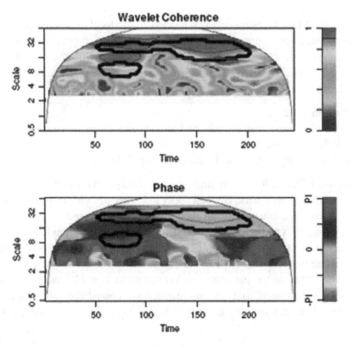

Fig. 2 Wavelet coherency analysis for two data sources, ED and IS

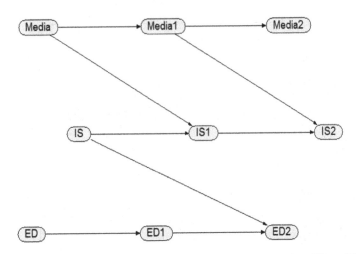

Fig. 3 DBN resulted from Bayesian networks learning based on media data, ED, and IS

we found different dependency relations between the two series by BNs structure learning. As the WCA suggested, we considered variations of candidate models with up to plus or minus 4-day lags. We also tried to train a DBN model with no phase difference between IS and ED in a DBN. The structure learning method also found that media reports data can lead the IS data by 1 day. However, this relationship only exists during the pandemic period in our datasets (April–December 2009).

We presented the Bayesian network models to the local experts in public health surveillance and asked them to assess the face validity of the dependence between the time series. The expert feedback was more in favor of IS leading ED. We experimented with four DBNs that correspond to the settings suggested by BN structure learning and WCA:

- ED leads IS by 2 days
- No phase difference between ED and IS
- IS leads ED by 2 days
- Media leads IS by 1 day and IS leads ED by 2 days.

We unrolled DBNs for seven time steps (weekly). We can treat the unrolled version of a network as a static BN and apply inference algorithms in BNs. We used cross validation for evaluation of all models. Four-fifths of the data were used for training and one-fifth of the data was used for testing. In each model, we provided the information for today's count on ED and IS and predicted the first to sixth next day's counts on both ED and IS. The second model works actually the best when it is trained and tested on the pandemic period (no more than 11% error in predicting ED). It should be noted that for all models we considered categorization for all variables. This includes media in {1–3; 3–7; >7}, ED in {0–100; 100–200;

Table 1 Performance of DBN models in predicting IS call volume, as measured by percent error

Model	% error					
	Day 1	Day 2	Day 3	Day 4	Day 5	Day 6
ED leads 1-day	19.49	21.19	22.03	26.72	29.03	29.9
IS leads 2-days	18.68	23.37	25.64	26.22	28.81	29.06
Media effect	18.24	24.21	26.72	27.65	29.31	32.59

Table 2 Performance of DBN models in predicting ED visit volume

Model	% error					
	Day 1	Day 2	Day 3	Day 4	Day 5	Day 6
ED leads 1-day	8.47	11.86	14.53	16.1	21.37	24.14
IS leads 2-days	8.47	11.02	12.52	13.33	13.56	18.49

200–300; 300–400; 400–500; > 500}, and IS in {0–100; 100–200; 200–300; 300–400; 400–500; 500–600; 600–700; > 700}.

Once built and trained, we use the DBN model to do real-time prediction through approximate inference in BNs. In this research, we aimed to learn DBN models that generalize well. The generalizability of a model is interpreted as the expected predictive accuracy for the next time steps. We evaluated the DBN model for prediction accuracy of important observations in time series IS and ED through cross validation techniques (Tables 1 and 2).

7 Discussion

An accurate measure of the incidence of infection with H1N1 influenza is critical for monitoring the progression of the epidemic and for guiding control measures. The direction de santé publique de Montréal collects data from multiple sources to describe H1N1 influenza infection and associated healthcare utilization. However, none of these data sources alone measure the incidence of H1N1 influenza accurately. Our results suggest that the integration of different streams of data together with Internet-based data into a real-time syndromic surveillance system may be a complementary tool for prediction of the impact of influenza during the pandemic period. This is in line with other studies, which have proposed that nontraditional data sources may be of significant use to augment current syndromic surveillance systems [7, 26, 27].

To the best of our knowledge, this study is the first to examine DBNs in the context of data fusion in an effort to provide an effective evidence-based surveillance tool. Although there exist dependencies between the media data series and the IS data, we did not see significant changes in the prediction results for IS. This can be potentially related to other factors which have not been considered in our model or solely related to the experimental setup we selected for these evaluations including the discretization levels of the media and IS variables and the information provided for reasoning at each time. The finer the level of the discretization, the less the stability achieved in the inference results from the network. Therefore, the results may vary with changing the categorization for the variables ED, IS, and media.

Our study has several limitations. Though one purpose of integrating the information in various data streams was to attempt to compensate for the biases of each data stream by incorporating information from other data sources, we must recognize that it is difficult to assess the extent to which the fusion of the data streams reduced bias. Misclassification errors could be present for a number of reasons. Although experienced physicians, nurses, and health coders provided this data, human error can still be a factor. ED and IS data are based on professional diagnoses, which are then converted to ICD codes. However, studies on the accuracy of ICD-9 (International Classification of Diseases, 9th rev) codes for respiratory illness have shown excellent specificity and moderate sensitivity, supporting their use in public health surveillance [5]. HealthMap data does not capture the sentiment of the reports, i.e., whether there were alerts of increasing incidence or epidemic/disease severity or if they were reports of decreases in incidence.

A variety of social, demographic, and environmental factors may contribute to patterns of influenza in general. This applies to H1N1 as well. For instance, the majority of 2009 H1N1 cases occurred in children, as the lack of cross-reactive antibody responses to 2009 H1N1 in these groups renders them more susceptible to infection. We did not incorporate such factors in this study. Also, spatial resolution and geographic information were not considered.

In terms of the utility of the DBNs in practice, exploring the stability of the relationship between these surveillance time series is important. It was noted in our results that the relationships appear more stable during seasonal influenza and less predictable during the pandemic. Adding media may help in the future.

Mathematical models predicting the course of H1N1 pandemic rely heavily on accurate estimates of the number of H1N1 infections during the first few weeks of the pandemic. Therefore, as a crucial first step to forecasting H1N1 incidence, the number of infections in the first few weeks needs to be accurately estimated. However, identifying the true cases of H1N1 and consequently determining the true number of infected individuals are difficult as some may have been asymptomatic or they may have had symptoms but did not seek medical care. Though we cannot determine the number of asymptomatic cases accurately, it is only possible to estimate the number of symptomatic cases through statistical models using data from existing influenza-like illness surveillance platforms. The estimates from these models can subsequently be used as inputs in mathematical models to predict the public health burden of the disease.

Although other data sources provide us with the prevalence of influenza, only the proportion of lab confirmed H1N1 cases can confirm the proportion of influenza that is specifically H1N1. We would like to evaluate the potential of the DBNs in incorporating lab confirmed cases to infer the total number of infected individuals.

8 Conclusions and Future Work

Monitoring health data is critical for detecting epidemics and for guiding control measures. In this research, we used data from multiple health-related sources to describe H1N1 influenza infection and associated healthcare utilization. We also explored the use of a web-based data source in public health surveillance of H1N1 pandemic. Evaluating the benefit of new data sources is an important step for improving public health surveillance. None of these data sources alone is believed to measure the incidence of H1N1 influenza accurately.

In this paper, we proposed a dynamic Bayesian network model for fusion of different heterogeneous data and to discover meaningful information from the relationships that these data sources exhibit. We showed how a DBN model can be used for generating short-term and timely predictions of real-time surveillance data.

We showed that even with only 1 to 2 days of data we can estimate future counts in the studied sources. These estimates will be useful in forecasting the spread of H1N1 influenza.

We will continue our investigations for choosing a better DBN structure. We plan to evaluate all lags (plus/minus) 4 and pick the one with the best prediction power. We did not consider the complete DBN model to predict the number of infected cases of H1N1 in this paper. After reaching a good DBN model for aggregation of data sources, we plan to extend the DBN model of observable data sources presented here to what is called an autoregressive hidden Markov models (AHMM) to contain the unobservable infected counts. We can then apply learning algorithms such as Viterbi and Baum–Welch on this hierarchical dynamic Bayesian network just as we can on HMMs to estimate the prevalence of H1N1.

Acknowledgements The authors thank the department of public health in Montreal for providing the data for this research and acknowledge the contribution of the members of this organization who participated in regular expert meetings. In particular, we would like to thank Lucie Bedard and Robert Allard for invaluable insights in the analysis of our results and in the preparation of this paper. This work would not be possible without the help and support from HealthMap group at Harvard University and from Annie Hoen for preparing the media data.

References

1. CIDRAP: WHO says H1N1 pandemic is over. http://www.cidrap.umn.edu/news-perspective/2010/08/who-says-h1n1-pandemic-over (2010). Retrieved on July 10, 2017
2. Gonen, M., Alpaydın, E.: Multiple kernel Learning Algorithms. J. Mach. Learn. Res. **12**, 2211–2268 (2011)
3. Stuart, J.M., Segal, E., Koller, D., Kim, S.K.: A gene-coexpression network for global discovery of conserved genetic modules. Science **302**(5643), 249–255 (2003)
4. Burkom, H., Murphy, S., Coberly, J., Hurt-Mullen, K.: Public health monitoring tools for multiple data streams. Morb. Mortal. Wkly. Rep. (MMWR) **54**, 55–62 (2005)
5. Reis, B., Mandl, K.: Time series modeling for syndromic surveillance. BMC Med. Info. Decis. Making **3**(2) (2003)

6. Heckerman, D., Geiger, D., Chickering, D.: Learning Bayesian networks: the combination of knowledge and statistical data. Mach. Learn. **20**(3), 197–243 (1995)
7. Espino, J.U., Hogan, W.R., Wagner, M.M.: Telephone triage: a timely data source for surveillance of influenza-like diseases. In: AMIA Symposium Proceedings, Washington, DC (2003)
8. Grein, T.W., Kamara, K.B., Rodier, G., Plant, A.J., Bovier, P., Ryan, M.J., Ohyama, T., Heymann, D.L.: Rumors of disease in the global village: outbreak verification. Emerg. Infect. Dis. **6**(2), 97–102 (2006)
9. Sebastiani, P., Mandl, K., Szolovits, P., Kohane, I., Ramoni M.F.: Bayesian dynamic model for influenza surveillance. Stat. Med. **25**(11), 1803–1816; discussion 1817–1825 (2006)
10. Brownstein, J., Freifeld, C., Reis, B., Mandl, K.: Surveillance sans fronti'eres: internet-based emerging infectious disease intelligence and the healthmap project. PLoS Med. **5**(7), 151 (2008)
11. Heymann, D.L., Rodier, G.R.: Hot spots in a wired world: WHO surveillance of emerging and reemerging infectious diseases. Lancet Infect. Dis. **1**(5), 345–353 (2001)
12. Maxwell, D., Chickering, D., Meek, C.: Finding optimal Bayesian networks. In: Darwiche A., Friedman N. (eds.), Proceedings of the Eighteenth Conference on Uncertainty in Artificial Intelligence, Morgan Kaufmann, pp. 94–102 (2002)
13. Grossman, D., Domingos, P.: Learning Bayesian network classifiers by maximizing conditional likelihood. In Proceedings of the Twenty-First International Conference on Machine learning (ICML'04), Banff, Alberta, Canada, p. 46 (2004)
14. Jensen, F.A.: Introduction to Bayesian Networks. Springer, Har/Dskt edition (1997)
15. Chickering, D., Heckerman, D., Meek, C.: Large-sample learning of Bayesian networks is np-hard. J. Mach. Learn. Res. **5**, 1287–1330 (2004)
16. Friedman, N., Murphy, K., Russell, S.: Learning the structure of dynamic probabilistic networks. In Proceedings the Fourteenth Conference on Uncertainty in Artificial Intelligence, Madison, Wisconsin, ACM Press, pp. 139–147 (1998)
17. Tsamardinos, I., Brown, L., Aliferis, C.: The maximum hill-climbing Bayesian network structure learning algorithm. Mach. Learn. **65**(1), 31–78 (2006)
18. Neapolitan, R.: Learning Bayesian Networks. Prentice Hall, (2003)
19. Pearl, J.: Probabilistic Reasoning in Intelligent Systems: Networks of Plausible Inference. Morgan Kaufmann, (1988)
20. Mallat, S.: A Wavelet Tour of Signal Processing: The Sparse Way. New York Academic, (1999)
21. Morlet, J., Arens, G., Foourgeau, I., Giard, D.: Wave propagation and sampling theory -Part I: Complex signal and scattering in multilayered media. Geophysics **47**, 203–221 (1982)
22. Grinsted, A., Moore, J., Jevrejeva, S.: Application of the cross wavelet transform and wavelet coherence to geophysical time series. Nonlinear Process. Geophys. Eur. Geosci. Union (EGU) **11** (5/6), 561–566 (2004)
23. Keissar, K., Davrath, R., Akselrod, S.: Time and frequency wavelet transform coherence of cardio-respiratory signals during exercise. In: Conference on Computers in Cardiology, pp. 733–736 (2006)
24. Li, T., Klemm, W.: Detection of cognitive binding during ambiguous figure tasks by wavelet coherence analysis of EEG signals. In: Pattern Recognition, pp. 3098–3101 (2000)
25. Torrence, C., Compo, G.: A practical guide to wavelet analysis. Program in Atmospheric and Oceanic Sciences. Bull. Am. Meteorol. Soc. **79**(1), 61–78 (1998)
26. Rowe, B.H., Bond, K., Ospina, M.B., Blitz, S., Schull, M., Sinclair, D., Bullard, M.: Data collection on patients in emergency departments in Canada. CJEM **8**(6), 417–424 (2006)
27. Wang, L., Ramoni, M.F., Mandl, K.D., Sebastiani, P.: Factors affecting automated syndromic surveillance. Artif. Intell. Med. **34**(3), 269–278 (2005)

Post Classification and Recommendation for an Online Smoking Cessation Community

Mi Zhang and Christopher C. Yang

Abstract There are an increasing number of health-related communities and forums developed on the Internet, where people discuss certain health issues and exchange social support with each other. However, due to the huge amount and loose structure of user-generated content in the health communities, it is difficult for users to find relevant topics or peers to discuss with. In this paper, we focus on an online smoking cessation forum, QuitStop. We extract user discussion content from the forum, apply machine learning technology to classify posts in the forum, and develop recommendation techniques to help users find valuable topics. Using text and health feature sets, the classifiers are developed and optimized to categorize posts in terms of user intentions and social support types. The recommender systems are then developed to make a recommendation of posts to users, in which the classification results are incorporated in the neighbor-based collaborative filtering approach. It is found that the combination of text and health feature sets can achieve satisfactory classification result. Integrating classification result could help relieving cold start problem in the recommendation. It can greatly improve the recall of recommendation when limited knowledge is known for a thread.

Keywords Smoking cessation · Social media · Classification · Recommender system · QuitNet

1 Introduction

With the development of Internet, a large number of health-related communities are developed on various social media channels. People discuss health issues in online communities without the time and geographical limitations. Social networking

M. Zhang (✉) · C.C. Yang
College of Computing and Informatics, Drexel University, Philadelphia, PA, USA
e-mail: Mi.Zhang@drexel.edu

C.C. Yang
e-mail: Chris.Yang@drexel.edu

© Springer International Publishing AG 2017
A. Shaban-Nejad et al. (eds.), *Public Health Intelligence and the Internet*,
Lecture Notes in Social Networks, https://doi.org/10.1007/978-3-319-68604-2_4

becomes an important feature of Health 2.0 [1]. Patients play a substantial role in their own health and treatment in the cyber environment [2]. They actively participate in discussions and interactions of online health communities.

In online health communities, users generate a large amount of text, which provides important health information and knowledge that are not available in other resources. However, due to the huge amount and loose structure of the information in online health communities, it is difficult for users to identify relevant topics or peers to discuss or interact with. It is import to develop data mining techniques to extract valuable knowledge and recommend proper topics for users. In this study, we extract user discussion content from a smoking cessation forum, QuitStop, apply machine learning technology to classify user discussions content, and develop recommendation techniques to help users find valuable topics. The approaches proposed in this work can be also applied to other health communities.

QuitStop is a forum on QuitNet website, an online intervention program of smoking cessation. A lot of QuitNet users are attracted to discuss smoking cessation issues and interact with each other in the community. It is found that abstinent smoking quitters are active participants of QuitStop [3, 4]. From our previous study [5], threads on QuitStop are assigned to different topics, and different types of social support are exchanged in the health community. In QuitStop and other health communities, users may have different intentions to participate in the discussions, and they may be interested in different types of social support. To recommend proper topics or threads for users, it is important to learn their intentions and interests. In this study, we first classify posts on QuitStop forum according to user intentions and social support types. Based on the classification result, we detect users' preferences to different categories of posts and utilize the information to boost traditional recommendation techniques, which helps to recommend proper threads for users.

2   Related Works

A lot of online health communities have been developed on different social media sites. Many studies use qualitative analysis to analyze the content of user discussion and develop different classification schemes [5–7]. Our previous research focused on user interactions of social support exchange and extracted five themes from messages on QuitStop forum, including offering social support, requesting social support, receiving social support, other activities, and irrelevant content [5]. Social support is "an exchange of resources between two individuals perceived by the provider or the recipient to be intended to enhance the well-being of the recipient" [8]. It is important for health intervention programs to help patients in establishing positive attitude and confidence. In online health communities, social support is exchanged between different users. Informational support and nurturant support are two main types of social support exchanged in online health communities [9–11]. Informational support offers information to assist patients in resolving health problems. Nurturant supports comforts and consoles patients, without direct efforts to solve the problems [5].

For online health communities, content analysis and classification of online health discussions are usually conducted by qualitative analysis with manual coding using a relatively small dataset. As a result, it is difficult to conduct this analysis on a large volume of data in real time. In this study, we apply classification algorithms to classify posts in QuitStop forum automatically. There are many classification models, including rule-based classification, Naïve Bayes, Bayesian Belief Networks, Support Vector Machine (SVM), Artificial Neural Networks, and so on. Classification is usually applied to online forums for question/answer detection and knowledge extraction. Different feature sets were constructed to detect and classify questions and answers in different online forums [12–15]. They are also used to evaluate the qualities of threads [16, 17] and analyze the completeness, solvedness, spam, and problem types of threads [18].

Although classification and other data mining techniques have been widely used in the field of bioinformatics, most studies applied them to biologic data that are well-defined and structured, like attributes of cells, genes, proteins, etc. [19]. Text classification is usually applied to academic records, such as documents in Medline/PubMed (A survey of current work in biomedical text mining). For social media analysis of health care, text mining and social network analysis are used to propagate infectious diseases with hospital records, predict pandemic increase with Twitter data, model hospital structure network, or analyze health social network for some websites [20].

In online health forums and groups, there are an increasing number of posts generated by users. However, it is difficult to detect the topics or themes from the unstructured data. Some studies tried to analyze the content of health posts on the web. Text mining is implemented to analyze posts of H1N1 [21] and sexually transmitted diseases [22] on Yahoo! Answers, as well as cancer blog posts [23]. However, these studies extracted concepts and terms based on standard medical vocabularies, like Medical Subject Headings (MeSH) resource. As a result, only medical concepts can be identified from the social media. Some important user interactions, like social support exchange, cannot be indicated from the vocabulary-based text mining. In this study, we classify posts on QuitNet forum with text and health feature sets without academic vocabularies. The classification result is used to improve recommendation.

Collaborative filtering is widely used in recommender systems. It is based on the assumption that users with similar preferences are likely to rate items similarly. There are two categories of collaborative filtering algorithms: neighborhood-based algorithms and model-based algorithms [24]. Neighborhood-based algorithms have the advantages of simplicity, justifiability, efficiency, and stability [25]. They extract user-item relations and construct user similarity matrix or item similarity matrix to make predictions [26, 27]. For two different items or users, the similarity between them is calculated according to the same users that recommend or rate them. The item (or user) similarity can be calculated by different methods, including correlation-based similarity, cosine-based similarity, Jaccard's similarity, etc.

[26, 27]. Based on the item (user) similarity matrix, different methods are used to predict users of an item, of which the most prevalent is k-nearest neighbors [25, 28]. Item (user) similarity matrix is usually sparse. Thus, neighborhood-based algorithms often suffer from the cold start problem for prediction [25, 28]. To address this problem, some studies select neighbors based on other sources like individuals' social network [29]. Improved methods are also proposed to calculate user similarity and build user matrix [30–32].

Some studies applied recommendation technology in online communities to predict discussion topics and participants. To predict users in a community, Fung et al. [33] adopted collaborative filtering approach and analyzed user-thread relations with Zipf's law and tf-idf. To recommend Twitter users to follow, Hannon built user similarity matrix for collaborative filtering recommendation and tried to boost the prediction by detecting user interests and matching their interests with tweets' content [34]. Yano et al. introduced topic models to predict participants of blog posts [35]. They combined topic models of LinkLDA and CommentLDA to generate blog posts. To predict participants of each thread in a dark web forum, Tang et al. developed a topic model UTD (User Interest and Topic Detection Model), to detect user interests and thread topics in online communities, which was used as a content-based approach for user prediction [36, 37].

In this study, we learn users' preference to different categories of posts and integrate the information into similarity matrices of collaborative filtering.

3   Research Goals

In our previous studies [5], we extracted five different topics from posts of QuitStop that indicate post authors' intentions. The topics include offering social support, requesting social support, receiving social support, other activities of smoking cessation, and irrelevant content. Moreover, two types of social support are exchanged on QuitStop, which are informational support and nurturant support. In this study, we develop classifiers to categorize posts and build recommendation models based on users' preferences to different post classes [38, 39].

We collect all posts and comments on QuitStop during 05/01/2011–05/31/2011 and 07/01/2013–07/31/2013. There are 5061 threads, 34,269 comments, and 1327 users collected. The classification and recommendation are implemented on the dataset.

3.1   Classification

Classifiers are developed to categorize posts of QuitStop forum. To construct training and test datasets to develop and evaluate classification models, we selected 375 threads from the dataset, which include 375 posts and 1365 comments.

The posts are manually classified as gold standard as described in our previous research [5]. 80% of the selected posts are extracted as training data and the remaining are used as test data. The training and test sets are randomly generated five times, and their average performance in the experiments is reported.

Two tasks are proposed for the post classification: classification of user intentions and classification of social support types. As mentioned earlier, there are five classes of user intentions, including offering social support, requesting social support, receiving social support, other activities of smoking cessation, and irrelevant content. Two classes are developed for social support types, which are informational support and nurturant support. For the user intention task, each post is assigned to one class. But for the task of social support types, the two classes are not exclusive, and one post could be assigned to either or both of the types.

3.2 Recommendation

In a dataset of N_T threads and N_U users, our goal is to recommend threads for each user to participate in (comment on). For a user u commenting on the thread t, we record the pair $\langle t, u \rangle$ in the dataset. A set of thread-user pairs could be constructed, which is denoted as TU. TU is randomly divided into a training set $\overline{TU}$ and a test set $\overline{\overline{TU}}$, such that $\overline{TU} \cap \overline{\overline{TU}} = \emptyset$ and $\overline{TU} \cup \overline{\overline{TU}} = TU$. Given $\overline{TU}$ known, for a user i in the dataset, we recommend him/her a thread set T_i with the size of K. For a thread $j \in T_i$, $j \notin \overline{TU}$. The top-K recall in $\overline{\overline{TU}}$ is used to evaluate the result. The recall of T_i for user i is calculated as $\left|\left\{ \langle j, i \rangle | j \in T_i \text{ and } \langle j, i \rangle \in \overline{\overline{TU}} \right\}\right| \big/ K$.

All posts and comments in the dataset are used for recommendation study, which includes 5061 threads, 34,269 comments, and 1327 users. Let $p = \left|\overline{\overline{TU}}\right| / |TU|$, which is the percentage of the test set. We set p as 30, 50, and 70%, respectively, and for each p value, we randomly generate five training and test sets for the experiments. For each experiment, the average result of the five sets is reported.

4 Approaches

4.1 Classification

We select different feature sets to build Naïve Bayesian classifiers and combine them through an optimization process. Experiments are designed to look for optimized combining weights for different evaluation matrices.

Feature Sets

Text feature sets and health features are constructed for the classification tasks. Text feature is widely used for classifications of forum data. On QuitStop, a thread consists of a post and comments made on that post. Texts can be extracted from different positions of the thread, including title, post, and comments. We built classifiers with text features at different thread positions, including title, post, and comments, and combine different classifiers linearly. To build text feature sets, we first preprocess raw text in different positions by discarding nonalphabetic content, removing general stop words, stemming, and lemmatizing with WordNet database. Then, term features are extracted and transformed to term vectors. As a result, each of the text feature sets is composed of a bag-of-words. On average, there are 2.6 words in a thread title, 72.6 words in a post message, and 21.4 words in a comment.

Some users provide their date of quitting smoking on their profile pages of QuitNet. Based on the information, we calculate quit status and quit stage for each user to build health feature sets. In our study, the quit status of a user in a thread is defined as the number of days that he/she has been abstinent from the self-reported quit date on the profile page to the day that he/she posts the messages. According to quit statuses, users of QuitStop forum could be divided into five quit stages [40]. Users with the quit statuses of 0 to 3 months are at Stage 1—early action stage; users with quit statuses of 3 to 6 months are at Stage 2—late action stage; users at Stage 3, early maintenance stage, are those who have been quitted for 6 months to 2 years; those with quit statuses of 2 years to 5 years are at Stage 4—late maintenance stage; and those who have been abstinent for more than 5 years are at Stage 5, which means that they have completed smoking cessation. Four different health feature sets are constructed: (1) PA status—quit status of the post author; (2) PA stage—quit stage of the post author; (3) CA status—the average value of quit statuses of all comment authors for corresponding post; and (4) CA stage—the quit stage distribution of all comment authors. We develop classifiers based on each of the feature sets, and combine them with the text classifiers.

Classification Model

For each classification task, we built Naïve Bayesian model based on different text and health feature sets, respectively. Then, different classifiers are combined and optimized. Given a post, Naïve Bayesian model calculates the probabilities of different classes that the post belongs to. For text feature sets and the health feature sets of quit stages, the Naïve Bayesian models are built on multinomial distribution. For the two feature sets of quit statuses, Naïve Bayesian models are implemented with a Gaussian distribution. For the task of intention classification, a post is assigned to a class with the highest probability. For the classification task of social support types, the two classes are not exclusive. Different binary classifiers are built separately for the two types of social support.

In the experiments, we develop classifiers on different feature sets, and then the classifiers are linearly combined with an optimization process. Precision, recall, and F1 score are used as evaluation indicators, and they are regarded as optimization goals to combine the classifiers. For each of the classification tasks, we first develop text classifiers on title, post, and comment feature sets, respectively. Then, the three classifiers are linearly combined to develop an optimized text classifier. Classifiers on different health feature sets are separately developed. Each of them is combined with the optimized text classifier. To combine n classifiers, let $P_j(c_i|X)$ denote the probability of message X belonging to the class c_i calculated by the jth classifier, we calculate the logarithms of probabilities and linearly combine them by

$$L(c_i|X) = \sum_{j=1}^{n} w_j * Log(P_j(c_i|X)),$$ (1)

where w_j is the weight for the jth classifier for combination, and $Log(V)$ is the logarithm value of V. For each of the k classes, $L(c_i|X)$ is calculated by Formula (1), and the message X is assigned to the class with the highest value of $L(c_i|X)$.

A genetic algorithm is developed to calculate combination weights in Formula (1). Each weight is set as a float between 0 and 1. Precision, recall, and F1 score are optimization goals in different experiments. At the initial stage of the genetic algorithm, 10 different weight combinations are randomly generated. Then, the population is expanded iteratively for 100 generations. In the genetic algorithm, BLX-α technique is used for crossover with the crossover probability of 0.75. Gaussian mutation technique is used with the mutation probability of 0.015.

4.2 Recommendation

Collaborative Filtering (CF) is the most widely used recommendation technique in practice. In this study, we apply classification result to improve CF methods in user recommendation.

Neighbor-Based Collaborative Filtering

Neighbor-based CF method is used as a baseline in this study. Let A be the matrix with the size of $N_U \times N_T$, where N_U is the number of users in the dataset, and N_T is the number of threads in the dataset. A is a binary matrix indicating the participating activities in the training set:

$$A_{ut} = \begin{cases} 1, & \text{user } u \text{ comment on thread } t \\ 0, & \text{otherwise} \end{cases}$$ (2)

ST is a matrix indicating similarities between every two threads. It could be inferred from A with J. The similarity between threads t_1 and t_2 is calculated by Jaccard's index:

$$ST_{t_1 t_2} = \frac{\sum_{i=1}^{N_U} A_{it_1} \times A_{it_2}}{\sum_{i=1}^{N_U} A_{it_1} + \sum_{i=1}^{N_U} A_{it_2} - \sum_{i=1}^{N_U} A_{it_1} \times A_{it_2}}. \tag{3}$$

For all users in the dataset, we calculate the probability matrix PC based on the CF information. It indicates similarities between users and threads, which could be used to predict the probabilities of users' participation in threads. The probability of user u participating in thread t is

$$PC_{ut} = \frac{\sum_{j=1}^{N_T} A_{uj} \times ST_{tj}}{\sum_{j=1}^{N_T} A_{uj}}. \tag{4}$$

The probability matrix PC can be used for recommendation and prediction. To recommend threads for a user u, we select top-K threads from PC with the highest probabilities.

Integrating Classification Result

In the last section, we propose methods to classify posts on QuitStop forum from the perspectives of user intentions and social support types. It is supposed that users have different preferences to different categories of posts to participate in. To solve recommendation problem, we learn users' preferences of different post categories and used the knowledge to improve traditional CF method.

There are five categories of user intentions, including offering social support, requesting social support, receiving social support, other activities of smoking cessation, and irrelevant content. For a thread t, we can construct a normalized probability vector $LI^t = \langle li_1^t, li_2^t, \ldots, li_5^t \rangle$, where li_j^t denotes the normalized logarithm of the probability that t is in the jth category of user intentions. Note that LI^t is normalized that the sum of all elements in LI^t is equal to 1.

For a user u, we extract all threads in the training set that u participates in, and construct a normalized vector $LI^u = \langle li_1^u, li_2^u, \ldots, li_5^u \rangle$, where $LI^u = \frac{\sum_{j=1}^{N_T} A_{uj} \times LI^j}{\sum_{j=1}^{N_T} A_{uj}}$. The preference of u to the jth category of user intentions is calculated by the average value of the probabilities of all posts that u participates in. If u does not participate in any threads in the training set, all elements in LI^u are set 0.

The classification of user intentions is integrated to improve the prediction matrix PC in formula (4), which leads to a comprehensive prediction matrix P:

$$P_{ut} = W_{pc} \times PC_{ut} + W_{li} \times CSim(LI^u, LI^t), \tag{5}$$

where W_{pc} and W_{li} are weights above 0 to integrate classification result with the baseline method.

Toward types of social support, there are two categories of the posts, which are informational support and nurturant support. For the thread t, we construct a logarithm vector $LS^t = \langle ls_i^t, ls_n^t \rangle$, where ls_i^t is the normalized logarithm probability of t containing informational support, and ls_n^t is the normalized logarithm probability of t containing nurturant support. Note that the sum of elements in LS^t is not necessary to be 1, because the two logarithm values are normalized for different types of social support, respectively.

For a user u, we extract all threads in the training set that u participates in, and construct a vector $LS^u = \langle ls_i^u, ls_n^u \rangle$, where $LS^u = \frac{\sum_{j=1}^{N_T} A_{uj} \times LS^j}{\sum_{j=1}^{N_T} A_{uj}}$. The preference of u to each type of social support elements is calculated by the average value of probabilities of all posts that u participates in. If u does not participate in any threads in the training set, all in LS^u are set 0.

Similarly, the classification result of social support types is used to improve PC. In this case, the prediction matrix P is proposed:

$$P_{ut} = W_{pc} \times PC_{ut} + W_{ls} \times CSim(LS^u, LS^t), \tag{6}$$

where W_{pc} and W_{ls} are weights above 0.

5 Results

5.1 Classification

Classification of Intentions

To classify posts in terms of user intentions, we first develop classifiers with text feature sets of title, post, and comments. Then we use health classifiers to boost the text classifier. The result is shown in Fig. 1.

Figure 1a shows the result of intention classification with the optimization goal of improving precision. The most efficient text classifier combines title, post, and comments feature sets with weights of 0.700, 0.602, and 0.085, respectively. We apply different health feature sets to boost the text classifier and found that the classifier with CA status (the mean of quit statuses of comment authors) could improve the precision greatly. So, the highest precision is achieved when combining classifiers of title, post, comment, and CA status. However, the recall and F1 score cannot be improved during the process.

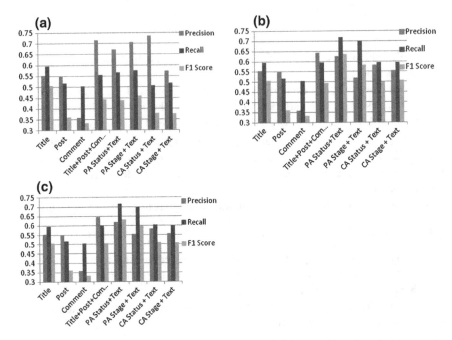

Fig. 1 Results of post classification of intentions: **a** optimizing precision; **b** optimizing recall; **c** optimizing F1 score

Figure 1b considers recall as the optimization goal. The text classifier based on title feature sets achieves the best recall compared to other text classifiers. To improve recall of the title-based classifier, adding PA status (the quit status of the post author) reaches the highest recall. During the process of optimizing recall, the precision and F1 score are also improved accordingly.

From Fig. 1c with the optimization goal of F1 score, the title classifier achieves the best F1 score among all text classifiers. Integrating PA status can greatly improve the text classifier, which is the same as that in the experiment of optimizing recall.

Summarizing all experiment results, the highest precision and recall are achieved by different classifiers. The classifier reaching the highest precision (0.715) combines features sets of title, post, comment, and CA status with weights of 0.678, 0.634, 0.362, and 0.711, respectively. The classifier that achieves the highest recall (0.719) and F1 score (0.636) combines feature sets of title and PA status with weights of 0.922 and 0.304. So, for post classification of intention, title is the most important feature that reaches the highest recall in text-only classification. Combining title with post content can achieve high precision. Adding health feature sets, including quit statuses of post author and comment authors, can help improving precision, recall, and F1 score.

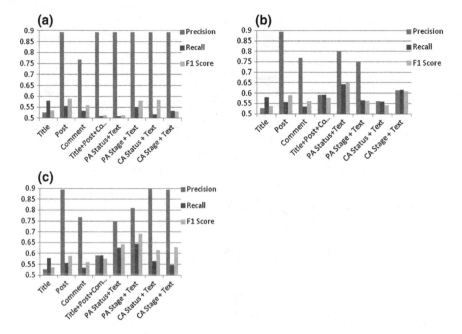

Fig. 2 Results of post classification of social support types: **a** optimizing precision; **b** optimizing recall; **c** optimizing F1 score

Classification of Social Support Types

The results of classifications of social support types are shown in Fig. 2. From Fig. 2a, the classifier only with post text has the highest precision. Adding other text features or health features could not greatly improve the precision. From Fig. 2b, combining title, post and comment can achieve the highest recall among all the text classifiers. The combination weights are 0.975, 0.038, and 0.108, respectively. Integrating PA status can boost the text classifiers. From Fig. 2c, post classifier reaches the highest F1 score compared to other text feature sets. Integrating PA stage can improve text classifier.

For all the classifiers, the one only with the post feature set reaches the highest precision of 0.894. The classifier that combines post and PA stage has the highest recall (0.645) and F1 score (0.692). The combination weights for post and PA stage are 0.155 and 0.997.

5.2 Recommendation

As shown in formulas (5) and (6), the classification results of user intentions and social support types are integrated to boost neighbor-based collaborative filtering.

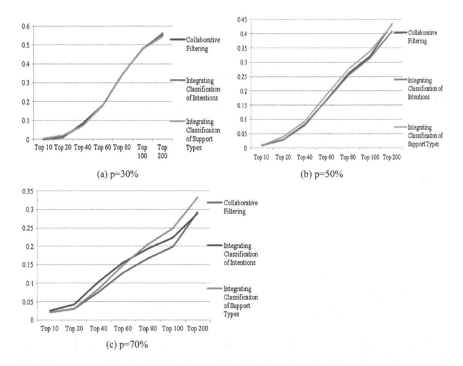

Fig. 3 Improving CF with classification results—Top-K recall with different percentages (*p*) of test sets

For user intention classification, we choose classifiers of title text and PA stage with weights of 0.8 and 0.2 to calculate LI^t. For classification of social support types, the combination weights are 0.9 and 0.1. To implement formula (5), W_{pc} is set as 15, and W_{li} is set as 1. For formula (6), W_{pc} is set as 5, and W_{ls} is set as 1. As mentioned earlier, we generate the test set and training set at different percentages. Figure 3 shows the top-K recalls with the baseline of basic collaborative filtering.

From Fig. 3, when the test set includes a small percentage of data (*p* = 30%), integrating classification results cannot improve CF method. However, with a higher percentage of test data (*p* = 70%), integrating classification results could apparently improve the recommendation. With the bigger test data, there is less information in the training dataset. It indicates that when a thread is initiated, and there are few participants known, we can utilize classification results to improve recommendation. After more people participate in the thread and we get enough information, the basic CF can work effectively for the recommendation. The classification result could be integrated into CF method to solve or relieve cold start problem.

6 Conclusion

In this study, we apply machine learning techniques to classify discussion content in QuitStop forum and develop recommender systems to recommend proper threads for users in the forum. First, we build and optimize classifiers to categorize posts on QuitStop forum in terms of user intentions and social support types. Text features and health features are constructed. Then, we use neighbor-based collaborative filtering to recommend threads to users and integrate classification results to improve the recommendation outcome. It is found that health feature sets can improve the basic text classifiers. Integrating classification result could help relieving cold start problem in the recommendation. It can greatly improve the recall of recommendation when limited knowledge is known for a thread. In the future, we would improve recommender systems with more content features to achieve better recommendation result.

References

1. Hughes, B., Joshi, I., Wareham, J.: Health 2.0 and Medicine 2.0: tensions and controversies in the field. J. Med. Internet Res. **10**(3), e23 (2008)
2. Wactlar, H., Pavel, M., Barkis, W.: Can computer science save healthcare? IEEE Intell. Syst. **26**(5), 79–83 (2011)
3. Cobb, N.K., Graham, A.L.: Characterizing internet searchers of smoking cessation information. J. Med. Internet Res. **8**(3), e17 (2006)
4. Cobb, N.K., Graham, A.L., Abrams, D.B.: Social network structure of a large online community for smoking cessation. Am. J. Public Health **100**, 1282–1289 (2010)
5. Zhang, M., Yang, C.C., Gong, X.: Social support and exchange patterns in an online smoking cessation intervention program. In: Proceedings of IEEE International Conference on Healthcare Informatics, IEEE, 2013 of Conference, pp. 219–228
6. Bender, J.L., Jimenez-Marroquin, M.C., Jadad, A.R.: Seeking support on Facebook: a content analysis of breast cancer groups. J. Med. Internet Res. **13**(1), e16 (2011)
7. Greene, J.A., Choudhry, N.K., Kilabuk, E., Shrank, W.H.: Online social networking by patients with diabetes: a qualitative evaluation of communication with Facebook. J. Gen. Internet Med. **26**(3), 287–292 (2011)
8. Shumaker, S.A., Brownell, A.: Toward a theory of social support: closing conceptual gaps. J. Soc. Issues **40**(4), 11–36 (1984)
9. Chuang, K.Y., Yang, C.C.: Helping you to help me: exploring supportive interaction in online health community. In: ASIS&T'10 Proceedings of the 73rd ASIS&T Annual Meeting on Navigating Streams in an Information Ecosystem, ASIS&T 2010, 2011 of Conference **47**(9), (2010)
10. Chuang, K., Yang, C.C.: Social support in online healthcare social networking. In: Proceedings of iConference 2010, 2010 of Conference (2010). http://hdl.handle.net/1860/3864
11. Eichhorn, K.C.: Soliciting and providing social support over the internet: an investigation of online eating disorder support groups. J. Comput. Mediated Commun. **14**(1), 67–78 (2008). doi:10.1111/j.1083-6101.2008.01431.x

12. Antonelli, F., Sapino, M.L.: A rule based approach to message board topics classification. In: Proceedings of the 11th International Conference on Advances in Multimedia Information Systems, 2005 of Conference, pp. 33–48 (2005)

13. Kim, J., Chern, G., Feng, D., Shaw, E., Hovy, E.: Mining and assessing discussions on the web through speech act analysis. In: Proceedings of ISWC'06 Workshop on Web Content Mining with Human Language Technologies, 2006 of Conference (2006)

14. Hong, L., Davison, B.D.: A classification-based approach to question answering in discussion boards. In: Proceedings of the 32nd International ACM SIGIR Conference on Research and development in information retrieval (SIGIR'09), ACM, 2009 of Conference, pp. 171–178 (2009)

15. Kim, S.N., Wangand, L., Baldwin, T.: Tagging and linking web forum posts. In: Proceedings of the Fourteenth Conference on Computational Natural Language Learning, 2010 of Conference, pp. 192–202 (2010)

16. Huang, J., Zhou, M., Yang, D.: Extracting chatbot knowledge from online discussion forums. In: Proceedings of the 20th International Joint Conference on Artifical intelligence (IJCAI'07), 2007 of Conference, pp. 423–428 (2007)

17. Weimer, D., Gurevych, I.: Predicting the perceived quality of web forum posts. In: Proceedings of Recent Advances in Natural Language Processing 2007 (RANLP'07), 2007 of Conference, pp. 1–6 (2007)

18. Baldwin, T., Martinez, D., Penman, R.B.: Automatic thread Classification for Linux user forum information access. In: Proceedings of the 2007 Australasian Document Computing Symposium (ADCS 2007). Melbourne, Australia (2007)

19. Saeys, Y., Inza, I, Larrañaga, P.: A review of feature selection techniques in bioinformatics. Bioinformatics 23(19), pp. 2507–2517 (2007)

20. Wegrzyn-Wolska, K., Bougueroua, L., Dziczkowski, G.: Social media analysis for e-health and medical purposes. In: Proceedings of 2011 International Conference on Computational Aspects of Social Networks (CASoN), 2011 of Conference, pp. 278–283 (2011)

21. Kim, S., Pinkerton, T., Ganesh, N.: Assessment of H1N1 questions and answers posted on the Web. Am. J. Infect. Control 40(3), 211–217 (2012)

22. Oh, S., Park, M.S.: Text mining as a method of analyzing health questions in social Q&A. Proc. Am. Soc. Inf. Sci. Technol. 50(1), 1–4 (2013)

23. Kim, S.: Content analysis of cancer blog posts. J. Med. Libr. Assoc. 97(4), 260–266 (2009). doi:10.3163/1536-5050.97.4.009

24. Breese, J.S., Heckerman, D., Kadie, C.: Empirical analysis of predictive algorithms for collaborative filtering. In: Proceedings of the Fourteenth Conference on Uncertainty in artificial intelligence, Morgan Kaufmann Publishers Inc., 1998 of Conference, pp. 43–52 (1998)

25. Desrosiers, C., Karypis, G.: A comprehensive survey of neighborhood-based recommendation methods. In: Ricci, F., et al. (eds.) Recommender Systems Handbook. Springer Science +Business Media, LLC, pp. 107–144 (2011)

26. Huang, Z., Li, X., Chen, H.: Link prediction approach to collaborative filtering. In: Proceedings of the Joint Conference on Digital Libraries 2005, ACM, pp. 141–142 (2005)

27. Huang, Z.: Selectively acquiring ratings for product recommendation. In: Proceedings of the Ninth International Conference on Electronic Commerce, ACM, 2007 of Conference, pp. 379–388 (2007)

28. Schafer, J.B., Frankowski, D., Herlocker, J., Sen, S.: Collaborative filtering recommender systems. In: Brusilovsky, P., Kobsa, A., Nejdl, W. (eds.) The Adaptive Web. Springer, Berlin, Heidelberg, pp. 291–324 (2007)

29. Zheng, R., et al.: Social network collaborative filtering. Working paper CeDER-8-082008

30. Huang, Z., Chen, H., Zeng, D.: Applying Associative retrieval techniques to alleviate the sparsity problem in collaborative filtering. ACM Trans. Inf. Syst. 22(1), 116–142 (2004)

31. Ahn, H.J.: A new similarity measure for collaborative filtering to alleviate the new user cold-starting problem. Inf. Sci. 178(1), 37–51 (2007)

32. Fouss, F., Pirotte, A., Renders, J.M., Saerens, M.: A novel way of computing dissimilarities between nodes of a graph, with application to collaborative filtering and subspace projection of the graph nodes, 2005. Retrieved on July 10, 2017. http://www.isys.ucl.ac.be/staff/marco/Publications/Fouss2004c.pdf

33. Fung, Y.-H., Li, C.H., Cheung, W.K.: Online discussion participation prediction using non-negative matrix factorization. In: Proceedings the 2007 IEEE/WIC/ACM International Conferences on Web Intelligence and Intelligent Agent Technology—Workshops, IEEE Computer Society, 2007 of Conference, pp. 284–287

34. Hannon, J., Bennett, M., Smyth, B.: Recommending twitter users to follow using content and collaborative filtering approaches. in: Proceedings of Fourth ACM Conference on Recommender Systems, ACM 2010 of Conference, pp. 199–206 (2010)

35. Yano, T., Cohen, W.W., Smith, N.A.: Predicting response to political blog posts with topic models. In: Proceedings of Human Language Technologies: The 2009 Annual Conference of the North American Chapter of the Association for Computational Linguistics, Association for Computational Linguistics, 2009 of Conference, pp. 477–485 (2009)

36. Tang, X., Yang, C.C., Zhang, M.: Who will be participating next? Predicting the participation of dark web community. In: Proceedings of ACM SIGKDD Workshop on Intelligence and Security Informatics, (1)

37. Tang, X., Zhang, M., Yang, C.C.: User interest and topic detection for personalized recommendation. In: Proceedings of 2012 IEEE/WIC/ACM International Conference on Web Intelligence (WI)

38. Zhang, M., Yang, C.C.: Classifying user intention and social support types in online healthcare discussions. In: Proceedings of The IEEE International Conference on Healthcare Informatics (ICHI), pp. 51–60

39. Zhang, M., Yang, C.C.: Classification of online health discussions with text and health feature sets. In: Shaban-Nejad, A., Buckeridge, D.L., Brownstein, J.S. (eds.) Proceedings of AAAI 2014 Workshop Proceedings of World Wide Web and Public Health Intelligence (W3PHI-2014), 2014 of Conference, pp. 24–31

40. Zhang, M., Yang, C.C., Li, J.: A comparative study of smoking cessation intervention programs on social media. In: Proceedings of SBP2012, Springer, Berlin, pp. 87–96 (2012)

Hashtag Mining: Discovering Relationship Between Health Concepts and Hashtags

Quanzhi Li, Sameena Shah, Rui Fang, Armineh Nourbakhsh
and Xiaomo Liu

Abstract Social media hashtags are useful in many applications, such as tweet classification, clustering, searching, indexing, and social network analysis. In this chapter, we present a Big Data mining technology on social media, and demonstrate how to use it to address the following three problems: discovering relevant hashtags for health concepts, discovering the meaning of health-related hashtags, and identifying hashtags relevant to each other in the health domain. The proposed approach is based on the distributed word representations, which are learned, by applying the state-of-the-art deep learning technology, from billions of tweet words without supervision. The experiment shows that this approach outperformed the baseline approach. To the best of our knowledge, this is the first study of applying distributed language representations to discovering relationships between health concepts and hashtags.

Keywords Hashtag · Health keyword · Hashtag recommendation · Word embedding · Distributed word representation · Tweet

Q. Li (✉) · S. Shah · R. Fang · A. Nourbakhsh · X. Liu
Research and Development, Thomson Reuters, New York City, NY, USA
e-mail: quanzhi.li@thomsonreuters.com

S. Shah
e-mail: sameena.shah@thomsonreuters.com

R. Fang
e-mail: rui.fang@thomsonreuters.com

A. Nourbakhsh
e-mail: armineh.nourbakhsh@thomsonreuters.com

X. Liu
e-mail: xiaomo.liu@thomsonreuters.com

© Springer International Publishing AG 2017
A. Shaban-Nejad et al. (eds.), *Public Health Intelligence and the Internet*,
Lecture Notes in Social Networks, https://doi.org/10.1007/978-3-319-68604-2_5

1 Introduction

A Twitter hashtag is a string of characters proceeded by the # character, and is used to build a topic community or as a descriptive label [1]. Usually, a hashtag consists of short, often abbreviated terms, and it is hard to understand its meaning without context or definition. On the other hand, given a keyword (concept), such as "cancer", one wants to know what existing hashtags are closely related to this keyword. Manually searching social media data to find hashtags relevant to a keyword is tedious and the result is not exhaustive. Similarly, given a hashtag, one may want to know what other hashtags are similar or closely related to it. A process of automatically discovering the relationship among concepts and hashtags is necessary. This paper presents such a method. This study focuses on the health domain, but the proposed approach is generic enough to apply to other domains.

Identifying relevant hashtags for health keywords can benefit the following health information related applications:

(i) Public health tracking systems based on social media can use relevant hashtags to increase its surveillance coverage. For example, MappyHealth (http:// nowtrending.hhs.gov), HealthTweets.org [2], and Crowdbreaks (http:// crowdbreaks.com) just track keywords and use tweets containing those key-words to do trending and other types of analysis. Due to tracking only key-words, these systems will miss many relevant tweets because lots of tweets contain related hashtags but not the keywords.

(ii) In a health social data search platform, users can search for hashtags relevant to a keyword, in addition to the keyword itself.

(iii) Hashtags can be used in automatic query expansion to increase the recall of a query, and it can also be used for query suggestion.

(iv) As topic surrogates, they can be used in tweet clustering and classification, and in social network analysis.

Given a hashtag without context, usually, it is hard to understand its meaning unless the hashtag consists of very explicit terms, e.g., #cancer. If we can show the relevant keywords for a given hashtag, it will greatly help users understand the meaning of the hashtag, and also potentially increase its usage. Similar to identifying relevant hashtags for health keywords, discovering health keywords relevant to a health-related hashtag also has many applications. For example, it can be used in retrieval system to expand the query if it contains a hashtag.

Identifying relevant hashtags for a given hashtag also has many applications. For instance, it can be used in the four use cases described above for identifying relevant hashtags for health keywords.

After we discovered the relationship between keywords and hashtags, and among hashtags themselves, we can use this relevant information to build a graph which encodes their relationships. Then based on that graph, we can discover the relationships between the health keywords. This will help to discover connections between the health concepts that are difficult to reveal by other approaches.

To identify relevant hashtags/keywords for a given keyword or hashtag, and use them in the aforementioned applications, one challenge is how to automatically discover the relationship with high quality. Most of the previous studies involving finding relevant hashtags focus on recommending hashtags for a tweet, instead of a keyword [3–6]. This chapter focuses on discovering the relevant information among hashtags and keywords, not for tweets, by utilizing distributed representations of words.

Distributed representations of words are also called word embeddings. A word embedding is a low-dimensional, dense, and real-valued vector for a word [7, 8]. They are usually generated from a large text corpus and the embedding of a word captures both its syntactic and semantic aspects. They help to learn algorithms to achieve better performance in Natural Language Processing (NLP) tasks by grouping similar words together, and have been used in many NLP applications. Traditional bag-of-words and bag-of-n-grams hardly capture the semantics of words or the distances between words. This means that words "pretty", "beautiful", and "train" are equally distant in spite of the fact that semantically, "pretty" should be closer to "beautiful" than "train". Based on word embeddings, "pretty" and "beautiful" will be very close to each other. In this study, the word-embedding representation model is computed using a neural network, and generated from a large corpus—billions of words extracted from hundreds of millions of tweets—without any supervision. The learned vectors explicitly encode many linguistic regularities and patterns, and many of these patterns can be represented as linear translations. For example, the result of a vector calculation v("Beijing") − v("China") + v("Japan") is closer to v("Tokyo") than any other word vector [9].

One advantage of using this approach is that it is an unsupervised process, and rebuilding the model to handle new hashtags and words is just a matter of ingesting new tweets to the building process periodically. It does not require any labeled data.

The major contributions of this study are as follows:

1. To the best of our knowledge, this is the first study that exploits distributed representations of words to discover the relationship among keywords and hashtags.
2. The proposed approach has practical applications in health social media platforms, such as HealthTweets.org, nowtrending.hhs.gov, and crowdbreaks.com. By utilizing this method, these systems can be enhanced by tracking-related hashtags, in addition to health keywords. In addition, they can increase the recall of searches by exploiting the relationship between keywords and hashtags.

In the following sections, we present related studies, the methodology, evaluation dataset, and the experiment.

2   Related Studies

Several health information platforms based on social media data have been implemented [2, 10, 11]. One of their main functions is the trending analysis of certain health topics by tracking health-related keywords. HealthTweets.org is a research platform for sharing the latest developments in mining health trends from Twitter and other social media sites [2]. MappyHealth.com (http://nowtrending.hhs. gov) fetches real-time data from Twitter associated with their predefined health terms and then analyzes those tweets and their condition sets for trending analysis. Crowdbreaks (http://crowdbreaks.com) is a crowdsourced disease surveillance system that collects tweets containing disease-related keywords. All these systems are based on keywords and do not include hashtags in their tracking terms or search indexes. In addition, they will miss many relevant tweets because lots of tweets contain related hashtags but not the keywords.

Previous studies related to hashtags mainly focus on identifying relevant hashtags for tweets, not for keywords. They exploit the similarity between tweets. Li and Wu [4] use WordNet similarity information to recommend hashtag for a tweet. Mazzia and Juett [12] apply Bayes' rule to estimate the maximum aposteriori probability of each hashtag given the words of the tweet. Zangerle et al. [6] recommend hashtags based on the well-known tf.idf representation of the tweet. She and Chen [5] treat hashtags as labels of topics and develop a supervised topic model to discover the relationship among words, hashtags, and topics of tweets. They also incorporate user following relationship into their model. Latent Dirichlet Allocation is used to model the underlying topic assignment of language classified tweets in [3] using a topic distribution to recommend general hashtags. Li et al. [13] incorporate topic-enhanced word embedding, tweet entity data, and learning to rank algorithm to recommend hashtags for a tweet. None of these studies focus on discovering relationships among hashtags and keywords.

A word embedding is a dense, low-dimensional, and real-valued vector for a word. In addition, it has been researched in previous studies [8, 9, 14]. One implementation is the word2vec from Mikolov et al. [9]. This model has two training options: Continuous Bag of Words (CBOW) and the Skip-gram model. Both models have been used by several previous studies, such as sentiment analysis and topic classification applications [15–18].

3   Methodology and Dataset

In this section, we first introduce the distributed representations of words, which are learned by a neural network, then the tweet dataset, and how to use it to build the vector model for this study, and finally the evaluation approach.

3.1 Distributed Representations of Words

Distributed representations of words have been used in other NLP-related applications, but they have not been explored in discovering the relationship between hashtags and keywords. A distributed language representation X consists of an embedding for every vocabulary word in space S with dimension D, where D is the dimension of the latent representation space. The embeddings are learned to optimize an objective function defined on the original text, such as the likelihood of word occurrences.

Collobert et al. [8] introduce C&W model to learn word embeddings based on the syntactic contexts of words. Another implementation is the word2vec from Mikolov et al. [7, 9]. This model has two training options, Continuous Bag of Words and the Skip-gram model. The Skip-gram model is an efficient method for learning high-quality distributed vector representations that capture a large number of precise syntactic and semantic word relationships. Based on previous studies and the experiments in this study, the Skip-gram model produces better results and here we briefly introduce it here.

The training objective of the Skip-gram model is to find word representations that are useful for predicting the surrounding words in a sentence or a document. Given a sequence of training words W_1, W_2, W_3, ..., W_N, the Skip-gram model aims to maximize the average log probability:

$$\frac{1}{N} \sum_{n=1}^{N} \sum_{-m \le i \le m, i \ne 0} \log p(Wn + i | Wn)$$

where m is the size of the training context. A larger m will result in more training data and can lead to a higher accuracy, at the expense of the training time.

Generating word embeddings from text corpus is an unsupervised process. To get high-quality embedding vectors, a large amount of training data is necessary. After training, each word (or phrase), including all hashtags in the case of tweet text, is represented by a low-dimensional, dense, and real-valued vector. Usually, the dimension size ranges from tens to hundreds.

3.2 Building Word-Embedding Vector Model

Dataset. Tweets used in this study date from October 2014 to September 2015. They were acquired through Twitter's public 1% streaming API and Twitter's Decahose data (10% of Twitter streaming data) granted to us by Twitter for research purpose.

Table 1 Basic statistics of the dataset

Number of tweets	198 million
Number of words in training data	2.9 billion
Number of unique tokens in the trained model	1.9 million

The basic statistics of the dataset used in this study are displayed in Table 1. Only English tweets are used, and about 200 million tweets are used for building the vector model. Totally, 2.9 billion words are processed. With a term frequency threshold of 5 (tokens less than five occurrences in the dataset are discarded), the total number of unique tokens (hashtags and words) in this model is 1.9 million. The word-embedding dimension is set to 300. The word frequency threshold and embedding dimension size are chosen based on our preliminary experiment. A larger dimension size usually will encode more syntactic or semantic aspects of a word, but with the cost of longer training time and more space to store the vector model.

Tweet Preprocessing Steps. Each tweet is preprocessed to get a clean version, which is then processed by the model building process. The preprocessing steps are as follows:

- All URLs are removed. Most URLs are short URLs and located at the end of a tweet.
- All mentions are removed. This includes the mentions appearing in a regular tweet and the user handles at the beginning of a retweet, e.g., RE: @espn.
- Dates and years are converted to two symbols representing date and year, respectively.
- All ratios, such as 2/9, are replaced by a special symbol.
- Integers and decimals are normalized to two special symbols.
- All special characters, except hashtags symbol # are removed.

These preprocessing steps are necessary since most of the tokens removed or normalized are not useful, such as various numbers and URLs, and keeping them will increase the vector space size and computing cost. Stop words are not removed, since they provide important context in which other words are used. Stop words are the common words that usually do not bear any content, such as *what, she, the,* and *from.*

Model Building. A word2vec [7, 9] implementation is used to train the word-embedding model. After the preprocessing steps described above, each of the 198 million cleaned tweets is processed by this word2vec tool.

Usually, a phrase has more specific meaning than a single word. Some health concepts are phrases, instead of single term words. To include phrases in the word-embedding model, the bigram and trigram phrases are first identified in each tweet before starting the word2vec model training process. This can be done using a phrase identify algorithm, or employing a data driven approach, where phrases are formed based on the bigram and trigram counts in the dataset, such as the approach used in [7].

After the model is built, it is saved as either a binary file or a text file, with each line containing the term (a word or phrase) and it's embedding a real-valued vector. The generated embedding model can be treated as a lookup table, and a term's embedding can be retrieved from this model. If the term does not exist in the model, then it returns null.

3.3 Identifying Relevant Hashtags or Keywords

For a given keyword or hashtag, we use cosine similarity measure (described later) to discover its relevant hashtags or keywords.

Find Relevant Hashtags for a Keyword. From the word-embedding vector model, retrieve the embedding vector for this keyword, and then compute the cosine similarity score between this vector and all hashtag-embedding vectors. Then the hashtags are ranked based on their similarity scores, and the top N hashtags (or based on a similarity threshold) are returned as relevant hashtags for this health keyword.

Find Relevant Keywords for a Hashtag. From the embedding vector model, retrieve the embedding vector for this hashtag, and then compute the similarity score between this vector and all keyword-embedding vectors. Relevant keywords are returned based on the similarity scores.

Find Relevant Hashtags for a Hashtag. Similar to the above two tasks, first retrieve the embedding vector for this hashtag, then calculate the similarity scores with other hashtags, and then the top ones are considered as the relevant ones.

Cosine Similarity Measure. Cosine similarity is a measure of similarity between two vectors of an inner product space. It measures the cosine of the angle between the two vectors. It is a judgment of orientation and not magnitude between the two vectors. Two vectors with the same orientation have a cosine similarity of 1, two vectors at 90° have a similarity of 0, and it is independent of their magnitude. The two vectors may have any number of dimensions, and cosine similarity is most commonly used in high-dimensional positive spaces. For instance, in information retrieval and text analysis, each unique term has its own dimension, and a document is characterized by a vector where the value of each dimension corresponds to the weight of that term in the document. Cosine similarity then gives a useful measure of how similar two documents are likely to be, in terms of their subject matter. In our case, each dimension represents one syntactic or semantic aspect of the term, and their values are numeric values. The two vectors have the same dimension size.

Given two vectors, A and B, the cosine similarity is represented using a dot product and magnitude as follows:

$$\text{similarity score} = \cos(\theta) = \frac{A * B}{\|A\| * \|B\|}$$

Updating Embedding Vector Model. After a vector model is built from hundreds of millions of tweets, we can retrieve the word embedding for any existing hashtag or keyword from this model. But this model does not contain embedding data for any new hashtag or keyword. To include new hashtags and keywords, we need to do incremental model training. This is more important for hashtags than keywords since there are many more new hashtags than new health keywords. The incremental training can be done periodically, e.g., weekly or monthly, and it is relatively fast.

Evaluation Method. In this study, we just evaluate the proposed approach of recommending (discovering) relevant hashtags for health keywords. The evaluations methods for the other two tasks, discovering relevant keywords for hashtags and discovering relevant hashtags for hashtags, are similar to this one. Since we did not find any previous study on recommending hashtags for keywords, we evaluated our approach by comparing it to the baseline system described below.

The Baseline. We define the baseline using the term co-occurrence method, which is a very popular approach in identifying the relationship between two entities. In this study, the relationship is defined as the relevance between a keyword and a hashtag. If the keyword and a hashtag appear in the same tweet, then they co-occur in this tweet. The hashtags are ranked according to their frequencies of co-occurrence with the keyword. For comparison with our approach, for each tested keyword, the top 10 hashtags are returned as the relevant ones. For each keyword, the whole dataset is processed to find its relevant hashtags.

The Proposed Approach. For each tested keyword, the top 10 hashtags were generated as follows: the keyword's 300-dimensional word embeddings were obtained by querying the trained model; the cosine similarity score was calculated between this keyword's embedding vector and the embedding vector of each hashtag in this model; the 10 hashtags with the highest scores were selected.

Comparing the Two Approaches. We selected 65 popular health-related keywords, such as flu and cancer, for the evaluation. To compare the two approaches, we took the top 5 and top 10 hashtags for each tested keyword and compared the two methods at these two levels. Each hashtag was evaluated by two domain experts, by assigning a score from 1 to 5, with 1 meaning not relevant and 5 meaning definitely relevant. The final score for a hashtag is the average of scores from the two experts.

For the annotators to evaluate each hashtag, we provided 15 tweets containing the hashtag to help them understand its meaning. The annotators could also check a popular hashtag definition website, https://tagdef.com, to find its definition, and use Twitter's search site to search-related tweets to better understand a hashtag.

4 Experiment

Figure 1 shows the comparison between the baseline approach and the proposed approach. It shows that our approach outperformed the baseline on both the top 5 and top 10 levels. The results are statistically significant at p-value of 0.01 using paired t-test. It also shows that when we recommend more hashtags, the performance between these two methods become larger.

Let's take the term "vaccine" as an example to see the top 10 hashtags returned by the two approaches. Table 2 shows the top 10 hashtags for term "vaccine". In Table 2, "Frequency of co-occurrence" is the frequency that a hashtag co-occurs with term "vaccine" in a tweet. "Cosine similarity" is the cosine similarity score between the word-embedding vector of term "vaccine" and a hashtag's embedding vector. A score of 1 means the two vectors are identical and 0 means they have no relation. Table 2 does show some difference between these two approaches. For example, hashtag #zmapp, which is a vaccine drug, is at top three using the proposed approach, but not in top 10 in the baseline list.

Fig. 1 Performance comparison between the baseline and the distributed word representation approach

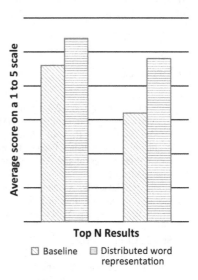

Table 2 Top 10 hashtags for the term "vaccine"

Distributed word representations		Baseline	
Hashtag	Cosine similarity	Hashtag	Frequency of co-occurrence
#vaccine	0.763	#ebola	1392
#vaccines	0.613	#vaccines	575
#zmapp	0.499	#vaccine	539
#influenza	0.477	#cdcwhistleblower	524
#getvaccinated	0.471	#vaccineswork	330
#rubella	0.46	#health	278
#ebolaoutbreak	0.459	#flu	277
#iamtheherd	0.459	#news	248
#flu	0.458	#hearthiswell	205
#ebolacure	0.458	#gopdebate	118

5 Conclusion

In this chapter, we described a new approach to discovering relevant hashtags for health keywords, relevant keywords for hashtags, and relevant hashtags for hashtags. It is based on distributed representations of words, which are generated by training on billions of tweet words. The experiment shows that this approach outperformed the traditional term co-occurrence-based approach. The proposed method is an unsupervised learning process and can be used in any content domain. To the best of our knowledge, this is the first study exploiting distributed word representations to discover the relationships among health keywords and hashtags.

References

1. Tsur, O., Rappoport, A.: What's in a hashtag: content based prediction of the spread of ideas in microblogging communities. WSDM '12, New York, NY (2012)
2. Dredze, M., Cheng, R., Paul, M., Broniatowski, D.: HealthTweets.org: a platform for public health surveillance using Twitter. In: Shaban-Nejad, A., Buckeridge, D.L., Brownstein, J.S. (eds.) Proceedings of the AAAI Workshop on the World Wide Web and Public Health Intelligence (2014)
3. Godin, F., Slavkovikj, V., Neve, W., Schrauwen, B, Walle, R.: Using topic models for Twitter hashtag recommendation. In Proceeding of WWW '13 Companion, pp. 593–596 (2013)
4. Li, T., Wu, Y., Zhang, Y.: Twitter hash tag prediction algorithm, In Proceeding of ICOMP'11 (2011)
5. She, J., Chen, L.,: TOMOHA: TOpic MOdel-based HAshtag recommendation on Twitter. In: WWW'14 Companion, 7–11 April, Seoul, Korea (2014)
6. Zangerle, E., Gassler, W., Specht, G.: Recommending#-tags in twitter. In: Proceedings of the Workshop on Semantic Adaptive Social Web (2011)
7. Mikolov, T., Sutskever, I., Chen, K., Corrado, G., Dean J.: Distributed representations of words and phrases and their compositionality. In Proceedings of NIPS (2013)

8. Collobert, R., Weston, J., Bottou, L., Karlen, M., Kavukcuoglu, K., Kuksa, P.: Natural language processing (almost) from scratch. J. Mach. Learn. Res. **12**, 2493–2537 (2011)

9. Mikolov, T., Chen, K., Corrado, G., Dean J.: Efficient Estimation of Word Representations in Vector Space. In Proceedings of Workshop at ICLR (2013)

10. Paula, M., Dredzea, M., Broniatowskib, D., Generousc, N.: Worldwide influenza surveillance through Twitter. In: Shaban-Nejad, A., Buckeridge, D.L., Brownstein, J.S. (eds.) Proceedings of the AAAI Workshop on the World Wide Web and Public Health Intelligence (2015)

11. Wang, S., Paul, M., Dredze, M.: Exploring health topics in Chinese social media: an analysis of SinaWeibo. In: Shaban-Nejad, A., Buckeridge, D.L., Brownstein, J.S. (eds.) Proceedings of the AAAI Workshop on the World Wide Web and Public Health Intelligence (2014)

12. Mazzia, A, Juett, J.: Suggesting Hashtags on Twitter, technical report. Computer Science and Engineering, University of Michigan (2009)

13. Li, Q.,Shah, S., et al.: Hashtag recommendation based on topic enhanced embedding, tweet entity data and learning to rank. In: The 25th ACM International Conference on Information and Knowledge Management (CIKM 2016), IN, Indianapolis (2016)

14. Socher, R., Perelygin, A., Wu, J., Chuang, J., Manning, C., Ng, A., Potts, C.: Recursive deep models for semantic compositionality over a sentiment treebank. EMNLP (2014)

15. Maas, A., Daly, R., Pham, P., Huang, D., Ng, A., Potts, C.: Learning word vectors for sentiment analysis, In Proceedings of the 49th Annual Meeting of the Association for Computational Linguistics: Human Language Technologies (2012)

16. Matt, T.: Document classification by inversion of distributed language representations. In: 53th ACL Conference, pp. 45–49, July 26–31, Beijing, (2015)

17. Li, Q., Shah, S., Liu, X., Nourbakhsh, A., Fang, R.: Tweet topic classification using distributed language representations. In: The 2016 IEEE/WIC/ACM International Conference on Web Intelligence (WI 2016). Omaha, NB (2016)

18. Tang, D., Wei, F., Yang, Y., Zhou, M., Liu, T., Qin, B.: Learning sentiment-specific word embedding for twitter sentiment classification. In: 52th ACL. Baltimore, Maryland (2014)

Studying Military Community Health, Well-Being, and Discourse Through the Social Media Lens

Umashanthi Pavalanathan, Vivek Datla, Svitlana Volkova, Lauren Charles-Smith, Meg Pirrung, Josh Harrison, Alan Chappell and Courtney D. Corley

Abstract Social media can provide a resource for characterizing communities and targeted populations through activities and content shared online. For instance, studying the armed forces' use of social media may provide insights into their health and well-being. In this paper, we address three broad research questions: (1) How do military populations use social media? (2) What topics do military users discuss in social media? (3) Do military users talk about health and well-being differently than civilians? Military Twitter users were identified through keywords in the profile description of users who posted geo-tagged tweets at military installations. These military tweets were compared with the tweets from remaining population. Our analysis indicates that military users talk more about military related responsibilities and events, whereas nonmilitary users talk more about school, work, and leisure activities. A significant difference in online content

---

U. Pavalanathan (✉)
Georgia Institute of Technology, Atlanta, GA, USA
e-mail: umashanthi@gatech.edu

V. Datla · S. Volkova · L. Charles-Smith · M. Pirrung · J. Harrison · A. Chappell
C.D. Corley
Pacific Northwest National Laboratory, Richland, WA, USA
e-mail: vivek.datla@pnnl.gov

S. Volkova
e-mail: svitlana.volkova@pnnl.gov

L. Charles-Smith
e-mail: lauren.charlesmith@pnnl.gov

M. Pirrung
e-mail: meg.pirrung@pnnl.gov

J. Harrison
e-mail: Josh.Harrison@pnnl.gov

A. Chappell
e-mail: Alan.Chappell@pnnl.gov

C.D. Corley
e-mail: court@pnnl.gov

© Springer International Publishing AG 2017
A. Shaban-Nejad et al. (eds.), *Public Health Intelligence and the Internet*,
Lecture Notes in Social Networks, https://doi.org/10.1007/978-3-319-68604-2_6

generated by both populations was identified, involving sentiment, health, language, and social media features.

Keywords Social media analytics · Sentiment analysis · Well-being · Healthcare analytics

1 Introduction

Social media has become a resource for studying different social, emotional, health, and economic conditions of communities through their online activities and shared content. Recently, there have been studies that seek to understand the emotions and behavior in different groups of people through their social media footprints [1, 2]. Other studies aim to investigate social issues and phenomena existing in communities through their online activities [3, 4].

Social media platforms, such as Twitter, contain publicly available information that provides a resource for potential identification of subpopulations and communities [1, 2, 4]. Applying machine learning and natural language processing techniques to social media content generated by military populations creates a potential to identify, characterize, and monitor their health and well-being. For instance, recent studies used signals from social media to study subpopulations online with the goal of detecting food poisoning within certain subpopulations and geographic regions [5], and identifying subpopulations of smokers and drug addicts [6].

Military service type (e.g., Army, Navy, Marine, Air Force, Active Duty, Reserves, and Veterans) may play a role in the health and well-being of military personnel, including the development of specific health conditions. Boehmer et al. studied the association between military service and health-related quality of life, using a population-based sample of adults in the US. They found that the active-duty population had more health complaints than either reserve or veteran populations [7].

In this work, we aim to understand the differences in online behavior and content produced by military populations, which share common characteristics, such as location, work, and culture, and compare them with nonmilitary populations. Specifically, the goal of this paper is to qualitatively and quantitatively estimate language variations and differences in communication behavior across these two populations.

Understanding social media activities and discourse of military populations may help decision makers gain real-time insights into their mental health, including social and emotional stressors, and other health-related issues of the military population through a minimally invasive and economic approach. Public health researchers and authorities could use the proposed methods to identify targeted populations quickly and distribute resources effectively.

Next, we list our research questions, provide some background, and describe our data and methods for identifying military users on Twitter. Then, we present our analysis and results. We conclude with a discussion of the implications of our findings.

2 Research Questions

Our motivation to study social media activities and discourse of military populations is to better understand their online social interactions and help to identify issues specific to military populations. Overall, we are interested in answering the leading broad questions by addressing the following finer research questions.

- How does the military population use social media?

  - RQ1: What are the differences in tweeting behavior between military and nonmilitary (control) populations?

- What do military users discuss in social media?

  - RQ2: What are the linguistic differences between the content produced by the military versus nonmilitary (control) populations?
  - RQ3: What are the seasonal trends of sentiment expressed in military and control tweets?
  - RQ4: What kind of topics do people in the military and nonmilitary (control) populations talk about on social media?

- Do military users talk about health differently than others?

  - RQ5: Are there any differences in the discourse of health-related topics by the military population compared to the control?

3 Background and Related Work

In this section, we first provide a background and summary of prior research about the US military population. Then, we briefly discuss prior work on understanding different populations through social media data.

3.1 Characteristics of the US Military Population

The US military consists of active-duty forces (Army, Air Force, Marine Corps, and Navy) and supporting groups (National Guard, Military Reserves, and Coast

Guard). Within the US, armed forces density varies by state; Texas, California, North Carolina, and Virginia have the highest concentrations [8].

In active duty and the reserves, individuals sign up for a specific length of duty and leave service or retire after that term. Three-quarters of the military population is less than 40 years old, and half of the active duty enlisted personnel are less than 25 years old. More than half of the military personnel are married, and 73% of married personnel have children [9]. The military population is diverse, without discrimination of sex, race, or native language. A unique characteristic of the military lifestyle is the frequent relocation of personnel and their families. The military is vulnerable to physical and mental health problems with nearly 18% of active-duty deaths caused by illness, and more than 10% of deaths are caused by suicides [8].

3.2 Studies of Military Populations

Since the US armed forces changed from drafting to enlistment in 1973, sociologists have debated whether to study the military as an institution or an occupation [10]. In general, the military is becoming oriented as a profession yet the military retains institutional features [10]. The US military population reflects America's racial, ethnic, religious, and socioeconomic diversity [8], however, their military status unifies them as a unique subpopulation.

3.3 Understanding Populations Through Social Media

As more and more users adopt social media, recent studies have attempted to use social media data to understand different subpopulations. Geo-tagged social media data is being used to identify populations in specific geographical neighborhoods and urban areas [3, 4]. Another body of work investigates specific demographic groups such as new mothers [2], fathers [1], and mothers using anonymous social media platforms [11]. These studies use social media profile information to identify users belonging to specific demographic groups or use forums to recruit subjects.

In line with recent research, we seek to study the US military population through the lens of their online social media activities, particularly through Twitter.

4   Data

Identifying subpopulations in social media with certain common characteristics (e.g., profession or location) is a challenging task. For our study, the data collection problem entailed differentiating public social media data from the military population and the surrounding civilian population.

Table 1 Military locations $L_1...L_6$ and the corresponding number of users sampled for both military and control populations together

L_1	L_2	L_3	L_4	L_5	L_6
4246	1040	1538	1372	1720	926

The total number of users sampled across six locations is 10,814

Our initial dataset includes nearly 200 million geo-tagged tweets from November 2011 to June 2015 that originated within a 25-mile radius of 31 US military base locations globally. We used this historical dataset to build a lexicon to identify and sample users who are likely to belong to the military population.

For our analysis, we choose six different US military installations located in three states in the continental US (Table 1). We chose locations that have a high ratio of military to surrounding population. For each of these states, we chose one control location that is at least 50 miles away from any military facility, and it was assumed that at this distance the users are less likely to belong to the military population. From tweets that originated within a 25-mile radius of military facilities, we sampled users who were likely to belong to the military population using the methodology explained in the next subsection. We sampled the same number of users from nonmilitary locations for our control dataset. In this manner, we collected up to 3200 of the most recent tweets (in June 2015) per user in the military and control samples. Note that this timeline dataset contains anonymized tweets with and without geographic coordinates.

4.1 Data Anonymization

We followed a rigorous data anonymizing procedure to ensure the privacy of all Twitter users. The data collected from a social media vendor and through querying the Twitter API was anonymized specifically for usernames, userids, and tweetids. This data was fed into an ElasticSearch engine where it was encrypted using the state-of-art encryption algorithms. Our analysis is based only on completely anonymized data and findings are reported on an abstract, aggregate level. Below is the detailed description of our sampling and data collection procedures.

4.2 Sampling Military Users on Twitter

While studying social media activities and content shared by the military population, our first challenge was in sampling Twitter users who are likely to belong to the military. Military population includes individuals who are on active duty, their family members, and veterans. The standard practice in identifying specific events or users in social media is to search for specific terms or hashtags in the tweets

Table 2 Example keywords used to identify military users

Group	Keywords
Active duty	Military, national guard, usmc, corporal, sergeant major, hospitalman, sailor, usaf
Family	Army wife, usnspouse, military girl, navygirlfriend, army brat, airforce wife
Veteran	Veteran, usnveteran, retired army, ex navy

[12, 13]. This approach was not appropriate for our experiments because we were interested in analyzing the content itself; extracting tweets with such keywords would bias our content analysis.

Another approach often used to identify specific users on social media is to use a database or web listings of users belonging to specific groups (e.g., an online listing of Twitter handles of journalists, used in [14]). However, to the best of our knowledge, there are no such listings available specifically for military users. Extracting tweet handles for some military organizations from their websites (e.g., @USArmyReserve, @camp_Lejeune, and @Military1Source) provided a way to identify only a small subset of military users. Therefore, we devised an approach for discovering potential military user Twitter accounts based on publicly provided content in the profile description.

To gather tweets that have a high likelihood of being posted by someone in the military, we extracted tweets that originated within a 0.5-mile radius from military base locations. These locations were selected based on the highest percentage of military-to-surrounding population ratio obtained from publicly available data.[1] The rationale for choosing a 0.5-mile radius was two-fold; it restricted the area and increased the probability of obtaining tweets from military users, and the resulting number of users per area is nearly 1000, which is a manageable size for faster annotation. Expert annotators classified profile descriptions of these anonymized users and the list of keywords extracted from the classified profile descriptions are shown in Table 2.

To sample Twitter users who are likely the military population, we extracted tweets from a 25-mile radius of the facilities in chosen military locations, and filtered tweets having most of the keywords from our lexicon in their profile description. Because we used both the geo-location and the appearance of keywords in the profile description to sample users, we expect our approach to perform better than the geo-location-based approach used in prior work [15]. For the control sample, we identified users from the control locations who did not include any of the keywords in their profile description. However, this control sample might include military users if they do not explicitly state their membership in their profile description. Timelines of the sampled users were collected and anonymized according to the description above.

---

[1]http://www.militaryinstallations.dod.mil/.

5 Analysis and Results

5.1 RQ1: Differences in Social Media Activities of Military Versus Control

To identify the differences in tweeting behavior between the military personnel (members and families in the military community) and control, we extracted the following measures: (1) size of their online social networks (i.e., the number of followers and friends), (2) interaction with other Twitter users (using user mentions as a proxy), (3) user's interaction with large groups of virtual communities (using hashtags as a proxy), and (4) ratio of geo-tagged messages to understand their practice of location sharing in social media. We present and contrast the mean counts that represent user activity and online behavior across populations in Table 3. We observe a high degree of variability among the military and control populations.

Twitter Usage and Frequency: We found that tweeting frequency is higher for the control population compared to the military. The differences in status counts and the number of followers per user are not statistically significant for military versus control populations. Military users write a higher proportion of tweets with geo-tags. Moreover, it has been reported recently that military personnel is allowed to use smartphones [16, 17], which have the geo-tagging capability.

The size of Social Network and Online Interactions: The mean number of favorite counts is higher for the control population and the mean number of friend counts is higher for the military population.

The mean ratio of tweets with mentions and retweets shows that military users interact less with others on social media using @-mentions and RT compared to the control, even though they have similar-size social networks. However, military users include more hashtags and URLs on average but less media content compared to the control population.

Table 3 Comparing mean values for user activities and online behavior across military versus control populations

Counts	μ_{mil}	μ_{con}	p-value
Favorite	1604.1	2113.8	***
Friend	663.7	498.2	**
Follower	955.9	976.0	
Status	8455.2	8268.4	
Tweet freq.	5.434	6.656	***
Geotag	0.155	0.138	***
Hashtag	0.216	0.186	***
Media	0.097	0.112	***
Mention	0.478	0.497	***
Retweet	0.200	0.239	***
Url	0.237	0.183	***

*** $p \leq 0.001$, ** $p \leq 0.01$

5.2 RQ2: Differences in Language Use Between Military and Control

Psychology literature suggests that language is a reliable way of measuring people's internal thoughts and emotions [18]. Hence, we focus on understanding military populations through the language used in their tweets. To identify the differences in the linguistic attributes between the military and control users, we first use a dictionary-based approach applying the psycholinguistic lexicon Linguistic Inquiry and Word Count (LIWC) [19].

Social media language, specifically in microblogs, is often found to be non-standard [20]. Although there are few recent works on normalizing techniques to convert tweets to a more standard language [21, 22], their performance has shown an only marginal increase in accuracy. Since these methods are at a very primary stage of development, we did not perform any normalization. Instead, we used an open vocabulary approach for extracting terms that differentiate the language of the military and control populations in complementary to dictionary-based (LIWC) analysis.

Differences in Linguistic Attributes

We used the psycholinguistic lexicon[2] to measure the differences in linguistic attributes. LIWC consists of several categories of linguistic attributes, such as linguistic or psychological processes, personal concerns, and speaking categories.

To measure the differences in LIWC linguistic categories, we aggregate all tweets per user, then count the number of LIWC terms in each category, and normalize these counts by the total number of tokens in the tweets written by that user. We compare the differences in LIWC terms for the military and control populations using an independent sample t-test. We report the results, showing only the measures that exhibit the same direction in the t-test for all military locations in Table 4.

Linguistic Processes: Our results show that the military population uses more *articles* (e.g., a, an, and the) and *prepositions* (e.g., to, with, and above) compared to the control. Military users talk more about others by using *third person plural words* (e.g., they, their) in comparison with the control.

Psychological Processes: Military populations talk more about work and financial issues compared to the control populations in social media, as indicated by higher mentions of *work* (e.g., job, majors, labor, and *money* (e.g., bank, income, and loan)) related terms. In all of the six locations, military users use more *home* (e.g., family, leasing, and housing) related words compared to the control, although none of the differences are statistically significant.

---

[2]Linguistic Inquiry and Word Count (LIWC): http://www.liwc.net.

Table 4 Differences in linguistic attributes between military and control populations measured using LIWC

Category	L_1			L_2			L_3			L_4			L_5			L_6		
	Δ	t-stat	p	Δ	t-stat	p	Δ	t-stat	p	Δ	t-stat	p	Δ	t-stat	p	Δ	t-stat	p
Linguistic																		
Article	5.4	16.0	***	1.3	1.9		2.2	4.2	**	1.7	3.2		1.6	3.2		5.4	7.4	***
Prepositions	10.0	16.1	***	1.5	1.3		3.3	3.7	*	4.1	4.2	**	3.3	3.7	*	9.4	6.8	***
3rd person pl.	0.3	4.0	**	0.5	3.0	***	0.1	0.7		0.8	5.8	***	0.3	2.62		0.2	1.7	
Phycological																		
Personal																		
Work	1.2	10.9	***	0.3	1.8		0.2	1.7		0.6	2.4		0.5	3		1.3	5.8	***
School	-0.3	-2.8		-2.1	-8.7	***	-1.7	-7.4	***	-1.9	-9.0	***	-1.4	-6.3	***	-0.4	-1.5	
Money	0.8	6.2	***	0.5	1.9		0.1	0.2		0.5	2.2		0.5	2.7		1.4	5.1	***
Home	0	0.3		0.2	1.2		0.5	3.1		0.2	1.4		0	0.2		0	0.1	
Death	0.1	3.7	*	0	0.6		0.2	3.4		0.3	4.7	***	0.1	1.4		0.1	1.2	
Religion	-0.2	-1.2		-1.1	-2.7		-0.2	-0.9		-0.1	-0.6		-0.1	-0.5		-0.3	-0.9	
Relativity																		
Motion	1.1	5.7	***	0.5	1.1		0.4	1.7		1.1	3.7	*	0.6	2.3		0.1	0.4	
Relative	9.2	11.5	***	1.2	0.8		4.7	4.2	**	3.8	3.0		2.3	2		6.6	3.8	*
Space	6.1	14.7	***	1.5	1.8		1.9	3.0		3	4.4	**	1.7	2.6		6.5	7.0	***
Cognitive																		
Inhibition	0.7	10.2	***	0.5	3.7	*	0.5	4.7	***	0.7	6.8	***	0.4	4.4	***	0.7	4.7	***
Causation	0.4	2.8		0.6	2.7		0.7	3.7	*	0.8	3.8	*	0.2	0.9		0.6	2.1	
Perceptual																		
Perception	-0.3	-1.5		-0.5	-1.4		-0.4	-1.7		-0.2	-0.5		-0.6	-2.04		-0.3	-0.8	
Spoken																		
Nonfluencies	0.1	3.2		0.1	1.5		0.2	3.5	*	0.1	2.4		0.1	2.2		0	0.5	

We only present linguistic categories which have the same directions across populations. $\Delta = (\mu_{mil} - \mu_{con}) \times 10^{-3}$ ($^{***} p \leq 0.001$, $^{**} p \leq 0.01$, $^{*} p \leq 0.05$)

Military personnel in certain locations use a significantly higher number of *death*-related terms (e.g., buried, died, and kill). Compared to control users, military users talk significantly less about *school*-related terms; they talk less about *religion* (e.g., church, mosque, and prayer) although the differences are not statistically significant. Military users in all of the six locations use *inhibition*-related words (e.g., block, constrain, and stop) in a significantly higher rate than respective control users.

Keyword Extraction

To find keywords that are specific for military and control populations, we extracted terms that differentiate language between these populations. We used a regularized log-odds ratio-based method [23], which compares the base word distribution of each group and outputs terms that are specific for each group. We show the top terms for the military and control samples in Table 5.

Looking at the top population-specific terms, we find that terms relevant to the events in military life (e.g., Semper [motto of US marine corps], barracks [buildings in military and facilities], boot camp, deployed, stationed, Sergeant, etc.) are more prevalent in the social media content of the military population. On the other hand, terms related to school, work, and leisure (e.g., ep [episode], tix [tickets], dorm, campus, Raiders [sports], Savemart, Blackstone [stores or businesses], Greensboro, Winston, Sanger [place names], etc.) are more prevalent in the control population's social media content.

We found that military slang words are widespread in the social media content of military users (e.g., oorah [battle cry of marine corps], hooyah [battle cry of the navy], chow [food], etc.); whereas the control users have widespread usage of Internet slang words (e.g., ep [episode], tix [tickets], ik [I know], tbh [to be honest]), and entity names (e.g., Greensboro, Fresno [place names], Bojangles [food chain], ttu [university], Raiders [sports], etc.). These results show that social media language of the military population is different from the control population.

Table 5 Keywords specific to each military and control samples, extracted using SAGE [23]

Military	Control
Deployed, sergeant, marines, Afghanistan, army, soldiers, usmc, stationed, marine, sgt, barracks, #marines, #navy, hooyah, ssgt, pas, oorah, napa, sempa, bragg, #semperfi, bliss, launch, veterans, ty, lejeune, bootcamp, corps, cammies, hooah, airborne, dam, okinawa, deploy, #veterans	pm, dorm, fresno, raider, #wreckem, lbk, tech, lubbock, frfr, burritos, pismo, ttu, ily, como, packs, Ep, shaver, rec, tcu, raiders, que, hp, bojangles, savemar, #texashtech, cheers, stock, campus, shaver

5.3   RQ3: Trends of Sentiment for Military and Control

Public opinions about real world events and concepts may change over time, and opinions are often expressed through social media. Temporal topical and sentiment analysis on social media data are active research areas [24, 25]. Additionally, the temporal topical analysis is useful for public health research, such as finding disease outbreaks through social media posts [26, 27]. To analyze the seasonal trends of sentiment, we created a temporal dataset by binning tweets from each month. Over a 12-month period, we compared same-user tweet content from military personnel and civilians who wrote at least 10 tweets per month. We used the VADER sentiment analysis library [28], which is a recent rule-based model for sentiment analysis with state-of-the-art performance. For each month, we obtained average scores for positive and negative sentiments of all the users and plotted the overall averages (Fig. 1).

According to the trend plots in Fig. 1, the sentiment scores vary across the months of the year for both the military and control populations. Overall, the military population expresses lower positive sentiment in social media compared to

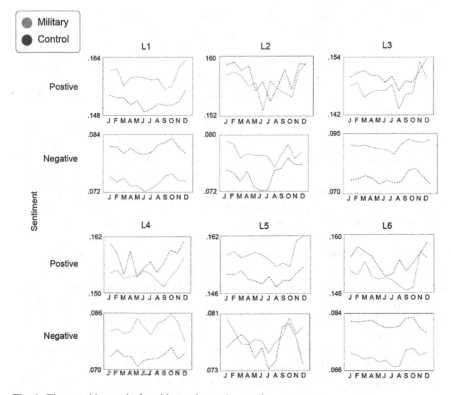

Fig. 1 The monthly trend of positive and negative sentiment scores

the control samples (except for the location L_1). Notably, the positive sentiment scores of the military population show an increased trend during the months of November and December, which is the holiday season in the United States (Thanksgiving, Christmas, and New Year).

Looking at the negative sentiment scores in the bottom row of Fig. 1, the military users express the significantly higher amount of negative sentiment in their social media content compared to others. However, the negative sentiment scores show a reverse trend for the two locations L_1 and L_6, which are located in the same state. Further investigation is needed to understand whether the location of military personnel affects their sentiment expressed in social media.

5.4   RQ4: Topic Variations Between Military and Control

Individuals use social media to report about their daily activities, life events, and opinions about various matters. The differences in the topics between the two populations indicate differences in social interactions and broad themes in their daily activities. Therefore, we aim to understand the differences in the language and the latent topics between the two groups.

Latent Dirichlet Allocation (LDA) [29] is a classic method for topic modeling. Topic models are based on the assumption that natural language texts are built using a small number of latent topics, and the words in the document represent those topics. LDA is a bag-of-words-based generative probabilistic model. The model builds on the words as observed entities, and then it learns the hidden (latent) topics by capturing intra-document statistical structure via mixing distributions of the observed words.

We implemented our topic model using the python library Gensim [30], which is based on online LDA [29]. After experimenting with several configurations, we determined that 100 topics are a reasonable number of topics. We combined all the tweets from a user and defined it as a document unit for topic modeling. We performed standard filtering and cleaning of documents by removing stop words and cleaning HTML tags, followed by lemmatization and stemming. As emojis (smiley faces, sad faces, and anger) are prevalent in tweets, and they are used to express emotion and other nonverbal cues; we included them in our data.

We trained the topic model using tweets from location L_3 (1538 documents in the training set, with a 50–50 split between military and control) with 100 topics and used that model to infer topics for the other five military-control pairs. Topics inferred from each document unit are averaged across all the users in the set to form two distributions for military and control. The averaged distribution across all the topics is compared against the military and control locations.

We selected the topics where control and military populations differ by more than 10% in the weight of their averaged distributions. The relative difference between topic distributions of military and control populations is shown in Fig. 2. The proportion of the average topic distribution of the military population is shown

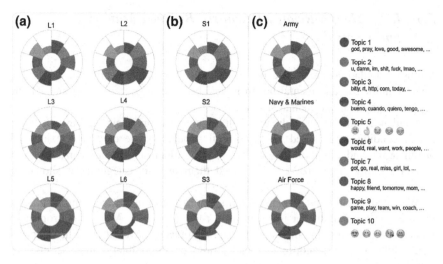

Fig. 2 a Distribution of topics based on tweets for military and control populations; **b** Distribution of topics based on tweets for military and control populations grouped by geography; **c** Distribution of topics based on tweets for military and control populations grouped by military service types. Colored area: military population, noncolored area: control population

in the colored area and the noncolored area represents the respective measure of the control population.

Figure 2a shows that across all the locations, profanity topic (Topic 2) is more prevalent in the military population compared to the control. Emojis (Topic 5 and 10) are highly prevalent in the tweets from the control population compared to the military users. Other topics do not show any consistent trends across different locations.

In order to understand the impact of geography and the type of military service (Army, Navy, Marine, and Air Force) on the topics, we look at further groupings. The military populations of states S_1 and S_2 use more Spanish words than the control, but in state S_3 the control uses more Spanish words than the military (Fig. 2b). We observe the same patterns of increased profanity topics (Topic 2) in the military population and emojis (Topic 5 and 10) in the control population when the populations are grouped by their respective states. When populations are grouped based on military service type, the Navy, Marines, and Air Force use less profanity compared to the control populations, while the Army population uses more profanity compared to their control group (Fig. 2c).

It is interesting to note that even a completely data-driven model such as LDA can pick up the differences in the social media content of the military and control populations. The differences are present in the topics showing emotional, daily activities, sports, and work-related activities. These findings are consistent with the results observed for our previous research questions.

5.5 RQ5: Health-Related Discourse Between Military and Control

Military populations are considered to be more vulnerable to infectious diseases, such as influenza, and mental health issues, because of overcrowding and a high degree of physical and mental stress [31–33].

To identify differences in the way military members and their families talk about health conditions compared to the general population, we created a lexicon of health terms and possible misspellings (e.g., "influenza" or "influlenza" for the correct spelling "influenza") and grouped them into six categories as shown in Table 6.

We calculated the total counts of terms appearing in user tweets and compared the average term count per token using a t-test (Table 7). After Bonferroni correction [34], we find that the direction and significance level of these health measures differ across health-related categories for the military and the civilian populations.

Overall, the mean frequency of health-related tweeted complaints from the civilian population is slightly higher than the military population across all health-related categories. These results are obtained through comparisons of military and civilian populations across different geo-locations and military service types. In Table 7, we show that civilians use disease-related words more frequently than the military.

Table 6 The example of health category keywords (ILI: Influenza like illnesses)

Category	Example keywords and stems
Self-related health experience	Suffer*, struggl*, fatigue, weak
ILI-specific symptoms	Fever*, cough*, shiver*, runny nose
Disease names and related terms	Influenza, sick*, flu, asthma
Health entities	Hospital*, doctor*, ER, clinic*
Parts of body and related	Lung*, throat, stomach, platelet
Non-ILI-specific symptoms	Breath*, diarrhea, dehydrat*, sneez*

indicates a regular expression, for example, fever indicates words that have a stem fever with difference suffixes such as fevers, feverish, and fevered

Table 7 Comparing the counts of health words for military versus control populations

Health category	μ_{mil}	μ_{con}	t-stat	p-value
Self-related health experience	3.04	3.35	−5.246	9.49×10^{-7}
ILI-specific symptoms	71.5	79.0	−3.701	1.29×10^{-3}
Disease names and related terms	1.06	1.17	−4.781	1.06×10^{-5}
Health entities	1.02	1.07	−1.576	6.90×10^{-1}
Parts of body and related	28.5	33.6	−5.134	1.73×10^{-6}
Non-ILI-specific symptoms	49.5	54.5	−3.623	1.75×10^{-3}

6 Discussion

In this paper, we analyzed social media data collected from military sites and corresponding control populations of users surrounding military locations. We explored the language and metadata inside the tweets from both populations in the following dimensions: behavior, language, and the discourse related to health topics.

Through the analysis of tweeting activities, we found that military populations use fewer retweets and @-mentions compared to the control group. As the usage of retweets and @-mentions are usually considered as a measure of social interaction on Twitter [35], similar to comments and likes on Facebook, these findings indicate that the military users are less interactive on Twitter compared to others.

We found differences in linguistic patterns of military users compared to the control: tweets from military users have a higher usage rate of articles, propositions, third person plural pronouns, and inhibition words; military users talk more about work and death, and less about school-related terms in social media. The increased use of articles suggests that military users use more concrete nouns, and they are interested in objects and things [18] compared to the control, while the increased use of propositions suggest that military population is concerned with precision [18]. Inhibition words are used to suppress strong emotions [36]. Therefore, increased usage of inhibition words by military users may suggest that they suppress the expression of strong emotional content in social media compared to the control population. Military specific terms and slang words are prevalent in the tweets of the military users while the control users talk more about school and leisure activities.

From our analysis, we observed significant differences in online behavior and discourse of the US military when compared to civilian users in social media. Below, we discuss the implications of our findings on life and health of military populations.

6.1 Implications for Military Social Life

Our study offers novel and interesting findings on social media activities and the discourse of the US military population. This is an early work toward understanding the role of social networks in improving lives of military populations. From our findings from RQ1, military populations have lower social interactions on Twitter when compared to the control users. This suggests that military users are socially less active than others in social media. Findings from RQ2 show a significantly higher usage rate of inhibition words, which suggests the self-consciousness expressed in the military populations' messages.

6.2   Implications for Military and Public Health

Our findings for RQ3 show significant differences in the usage of medically related terms between military versus civilian populations on Twitter. Overall, civilian populations tend to use more health-related terms (diseases, symptoms, etc.) than military populations. Although, we cannot conclude that military populations are healthier compared to the civilian populations, as further study is needed to explore the usage of colloquial language or military jargon instead of the standard disease terminology. However, the direction of the variables that indicate health-related terms shows that there are significant differences in the way military and civilian populations talk about health in social media.

The discovered health-related expressions of military personnel on Twitter suggest that it is possible to utilize social media content from military users to identify emerging health issues that are prevalent in the military population due to the nature of their job and living conditions. Faster and better identification of health-related issues have implications on public health.

6.3   Limitations and Future Work

First, we relied on social media content from Twitter alone to study our research questions. Using only one social media source is a limitation and future work can expand this to other sources such as Facebook and Reddit. Second, we relied on the geo-tagged tweets for the initial identification of military users. However, recent work shows biases in the geo-tagged Twitter data regarding text content [37] and suggests considerations of these biases when generalizing research findings. Third, we relied on geo-origins of the tweets, and keywords in Twitter profile descriptions to extract users belonging to the military, but better identification methods can be explored. Fourth, we did not take into account demographics for military and control populations.

There are several directions for future work. Complementing this analysis with an interview study about social media usage of the military users will help researchers and decision makers to understand the limitations in using social media among military personnel.

Moreover, linguistic differences between military and civilian users would enable the construction of classification models to automatically identify military users in social media. Expanding the analysis on health discourse and deriving cues about military health issues to predict disease outbreaks is another possible direction.

Finally, understanding the discourse of military when compared to the civilians helps to identify and prevent social issues affecting them non-evasively. For instance, differences in discourse between military and nonmilitary populations have been effectively used in other studies to identify emotional stress, depression, and PTSD-related illness. In future, we would like to study fine-grained emotional differences between military and nonmilitary populations over time, and model language variations among populations more effectively.

7 Conclusion

In this work, we studied language and online behavior of military populations in comparison to civilians within the same geographic region through social media. We observed significant differences in tweeting behavior between these populations. We further analyzed language inside the tweets and observed that there are significant linguistic differences in emotion and psychological words used between military and civilian populations. Finally, we found that there are significant differences in health-related discourse between the military and civilian populations.

Acknowledgements The authors thank Commander Jean-Paul Chretien, Aaron Kite-Powell, and Vivek Khatri, who were at the Armed Forces Health Surveillance Branch, Defense Health Agency, for helpful discussions on the research and experimental design of this study.

References

1. Ammari, T., Schoenebeck, S.: Understanding and supporting fathers and fatherhood on social media sites. In: Proceedings of the 33rd Annual ACM Conference on Human Factors in Computing Systems, pp. 1905–1914. ACM (2015)
2. De Choudhury, M., Counts, S., Horvitz, E.: Predicting postpartum changes in emotion and behavior via social media. In: Proceedings of the SIGCHI Conference on Human Factors in Computing Systems, pp. 3267–3276. ACM (2013)
3. Delgado Valdes, J.M., Eisenstein, J., De Choudhury, M.: Psychological effects of urban crime gleaned from social media. In: Proceedings of ICWSM (Apr 2015). http://www.aaai.org/ocs/index.php/ICWSM/ICWSM15/paper/view/10563
4. Lin, Y.R.: Assessing sentiment segregation in urban communities. In: Proceedings of the 2014 International Conference on Social Computing. SocialCom '14, pp. 9:1–9:8. ACM, New York, NY, USA (2014). http://doi.acm.org/10.1145/2639968.2640066
5. Harris, J., Mansour, R., Choucair, B., Olson, J., Nissen, C., Bhatt, J., Brown, S.: Health department use of social media to identify foodborne illness-Chicago, Illinois, 2013–2014. MMWR Morb. Mortal. Wkly. Rep. **63**(32), 681 (2014)
6. Paul, M.J., Dredze, M.: Drug extraction from the web: summarizing drug experiences with multi-dimensional topic models. In: Proceedings of HLT-NAACL, pp. 168–178 (2013)
7. Boehmer, T.K., Boothe, V.L., Flanders, W.D., Barrett, D.H.: Health-related quality of life of U.S. military personnel: a population-based study. Mil. Med **168**(11), 941–947 (Nov 2003). http://search.proquest.com/docview/217055081?pq-origsite=gscholar
8. Segal, D.R., Segal, M.W.: America's military population, vol. 59. Population Reference Bureau Washington, DC (2004)
9. Office of the Deputy Assistant Secretary of Defense: Demographics report (2013) http://download.militaryonesource.mil/12038/MOS/Reports/2013-Demographics-Report.pdf

10. Siebold, G.L.: Core issues and theory in military sociology. Journal of Political and Military Sociology **29**(1), 140–159 (2001)
11. Schoenebeck, S.Y.: The Secret Life of Online Moms: Anonymity and Disinhibition on YouBeMom.com. In: Proceedings of ICWSM (2013)
12. Cui, A., Zhang, M., Liu, Y., Ma, S., Zhang, K.: Discover breaking events with popular hashtags in twitter. In: Proceedings of CIKM, pp. 1794–1798. ACM, New York, NY, USA (2012). http://doi.acm.org/10.1145/2396761.2398519
13. Starbird, K., Maddock, J., Orand, M., Achterman, P., Mason, R.M.: Rumors, false flags, and digital vigilantes: misinformation on twitter after the 2013 Boston Marathon Bombing. In: Proceedings of Conference (2014)
14. Soni, S., Mitra, T., Gilbert, E., Eisenstein, J.: Modeling Factuality Judgments in Social Media Text. In: Proceedings of ACL. Baltimore, MD (2014), http://www.aclweb.org/anthology/P/P14/P14-2068.xhtml
15. Coppersmith, G., Harman, C., Dredze, M.: Measuring post traumatic stress disorder in twitter. In: Proceedings of ICWSM (May 2014). http://www.aaai.org/ocs/index.php/ICWSM/ICWSM14/paper/view/8079
16. Dave Lee North America Technology: US military approves Android phones for soldiers (2013) http://www.bbc.com/news/technology-22395602
17. Powers, R.: Can I use my cell phone during basic training? (Dec 2014). http://usmilitaryabout.com/od/armyjoin/a/basiccellphone.htm
18. Tausczik, Y.R., Pennebaker, J.W.: The psychological meaning of words: LIWC and computerized text analysis methods. J. Lang Soc Psychol **29**(1), 24–54 (2010)
19. Pennebaker, J.W., Francis, M.E., Booth, R.J.: Linguistic inquiry and word count: LIWC 2001. Mahway: Lawrence Erlbaum Associates **71**, 2001 (2001)
20. Eisenstein, J.: What to do about bad language on the internet. In: Proceedings of NAACL, pp. 359–369. ACL, Stroudsburg, Pennsylvania (2013). http://www.aclweb.org/anthology/N13-1037
21. Han, B., Baldwin, T.: Lexical normalisation of short text messages: Makn sens a# twitter. In: Proceedings of HLT-Volume 1, pp. 368–378. ACL (2011)
22. Yang, Y., Eisenstein, J.: A log-linear model for unsupervised text normalization. In: Proceedings of EMNLP, pp. 61–72. ACL (2013)
23. Eisenstein, J., Ahmed, A., Xing, E.P.: Sparse additive generative models of text. In: Proceedings of ICML, Seattle, WA, pp. 1041–1048 (2011). http://www.icml-2011.org/papers/534_icmlpaper.pdf
24. Diakopoulos, N.A., Shamma, D.A.: Characterizing debate performance via aggregated twitter sentiment. In: Proceedings of the SIGCHI Conference on Human Factors in Computing Systems, pp. 1195–1198. ACM (2010)
25. Mei, Q., Ling, X., Wondra, M., Su, H., Zhai, C.: Topic sentiment mixture: modeling facets and opinions in weblogs. In: Proceedings of the 16th International Conference on World Wide Web, pp. 171–180. ACM (2007)
26. Corley, C.D., Cook, D.J., Mikler, A.R., Singh, K.P.: Text and structural data mining of influenza mentions in web and social media. Int. J. Environ. Res. Public Health **7**(2), 596–615 (2010)
27. Culotta, A.: Towards detecting influenza epidemics by analyzing twitter messages. In: Proceedings of the First Workshop on Social Media Analytics. pp. 115–122. ACM (2010)
28. Hutto, C.J., Gilbert, E.: VADER: A parsimonious rule-based model for sentiment analysis of social media text. In: Eighth International AAAI Conference on Weblogs and Social Media (2014). http://www.aaai.org/ocs/index.php/ICWSM/ICWSM14/ paper/view/8109
29. Blei, D.M., Ng, A.Y., Jordan, M.I.: Latent dirichlet allocation. J Mach. Learn. Res. **3**, 993–1022 (2003)
30. Rehurek, R., Sojka, P.: Software framework for topic modelling with large corpora. In: Proceedings of LREC 2010 workshop New Challenges for NLP Frameworks, pp. 46–50. University of Malta, Valletta, Malta (2010). http://www.fi.muni.cz/usr/sojka/presentations/lrec2010-poster-rehurek-sojka.pdf

31. Gray, G.C., Callahan, J.D., Hawksworth, A.W., Fisher, C.A., Gaydos, J.C.: Respiratory diseases among US military personnel: countering emerging threats. Emerg. Infect. Dis. **5**(3), 379 (1999)
32. Pflanz, S.: Occupational stress and psychiatric illness in the military: investigation of the relationship between occupational stress and mental illness among military mental health patients. Mil. Med. **166**(6), 457 (2001)
33. Russell, K.L., Broderick, M.P., Franklin, S.E., Blyn, L.B., Freed, N.E., Moradi, E., Ecker, D.J., Kammerer, P.E., Osuna, M.A., Kajon, A.E.: others: transmission dynamics and prospective environmental sampling of adenovirus in a military recruit setting. J. Infect. Dis. **194**(7), 877–885 (2006)
34. Dunn, O.J.: Multiple comparisons among means. J. Am. Stat. Assoc. **56**(293), 52–64 (1961)
35. Macskassy, S.A.: On the study of social interactions in twitter. In: Proceedings of ICWSM (2012)
36. Rand, D.G., Kraft-Todd, G., Gruber, J.: The collective benefits of feeling good and letting go: positive emotion and (dis) inhibition interact to predict cooperative behavior. PloS One **10**(1), e0117426 (2015)
37. Pavalanathan, U., Eisenstein, J.: Confounds and consequences in geotagged Twitter data. In: Proceedings of EMNLP, pp. 2138–2148. ACL, Lisbon, Portugal (September 2015). http://aclweb.org/anthology/D15-1256

Towards Monitoring Marijuana Activities via User-Generated Content Platforms and Social Networks

Anh Nguyen, Hoang Pham, Dong Nguyen and Tuan Tran

Abstract Marijuana has been legalized for medical and recreational use in many states across the U.S. Despite some medical benefits, over the past decade, researchers around the globe have documented the health risks associated with marijuana use in both youths and adults. Monitoring and understanding the related concerns and activities of marijuana use play key roles in preparing and making appropriate policies for public health regulations. However, accurately and efficiently obtaining such information is very challenging due to the unique characteristics of the relevant users, where related activities are usually hidden or undercovered. In this book chapter, we discuss new approaches to reveal the related information of marijuana use in the community by exploiting information exchanged or posted in social networks. We show that data mining approaches can be used to shed some light on the hidden patterns and related activities of marijuana use from information collected in social networks (e.g., Craigslist and Twitter). Our approaches can be utilized as a new way for public health regulators to efficiently monitor and surveil-related activities of marijuana use.

Keywords Marijuana use · Attitudes and health effects · Marijuana surveillance · Online communities · Social media · Online behavior monitoring

A. Nguyen (✉) · D. Nguyen
Saolasoft Inc., Centennial, CO, USA
e-mail: anguyen@saolasoft.com

D. Nguyen
e-mail: dnguyen@saolasoft.com

T. Tran
Sullivan University, Louisville, KY, USA
e-mail: ttran@sullivan.edu

H. Pham
Piscataway, USA
e-mail: phamthaihoang.hn@gmail.com

© Springer International Publishing AG 2017
A. Shaban-Nejad et al. (eds.), *Public Health Intelligence and the Internet*,
Lecture Notes in Social Networks, https://doi.org/10.1007/978-3-319-68604-2_7

1 Introduction

Together with the fast pace of state legalizations of recreational marijuana, the number of marijuana users increases accordingly, leading to the high prevalence rate of marijuana use, abuse, and dependence. According to the National Survey on Drug Use and Health (NSDUH), in 2013, there are approximately 2.4 million persons older than 12 years had smoked marijuana for the first time during the preceding 12 months, and nearly 6600 people start using marijuana each day [1]. While the trend in substance consumption increases, the risk perception considerably subdues. In particular, the NSDUH data shows that the prevalence of past month marijuana exposure among persons aged 12–17 years increased from 6.7% in 2006 to 7.1% in 2013. On the other hand, the percentage who recognized prominent risk from smoking marijuana once a month decreased from 34.6% in 2006 to 24.2% in 2013 [1].

Although health risks associated with smoking marijuana is still debated [2, 3], some major studies have confirmed the adverse effects of the substance abuse, posing potential public health concerns. Depending on cannabis for long-term reduces educational attainment [4]. The addiction in some users increases the risk for psychosis disorders [5], alters brain structure and function [6], and substantially impairs the driving ability [7]. Additionally, research [8, 9] also showed a strong relationship between the use of marijuana with users' health harms including heart attack risks, lung irritants or a cough, mental illness, or birth weight decrease. Furthermore, data provided by the U.S. National Survey on Drug User and Health [10] indicated that youth with poor academic results were more than four times as likely to have used marijuana in the past year than youth with an average of higher grades. That said, marijuana poses considerable danger to the health and safety of the users themselves, their families, and their communities. Surveillance of actual marijuana demographics use and concerns would be very helpful for federal law and health policy makers to develop appropriate public health regulations.

The current methods for conducting marijuana use surveillance, for example, the one by the Centers for Disease Control and Prevention (CDC), fundamentally rely on traditional survey method. Specifically, CDC has conducted a national- and state-level survey called The National Survey on Drug Use and Health. The NSDUH has been carried out via household face-to-face interviews, and the result is published only once a year. Obviously, this method is time-consuming, labor-intensive, as well as expensive. This method typically results in few months reporting lag and covers a small percentage of the whole population. Furthermore, this approach may not be able to detect the actual level of marijuana usage as the interviewees may hide the truth of their marijuana use [11]. Therefore, it is important to develop an effective, accurate method to monitor and detect marijuana use in the community.

Recently, with the popularity of social networks such as Twitter, Facebook, Instagram, or Snapchat, the public health surveillance based on social media information is very appealing. This emerging approach provides several advantages compared with the existing approaches:

- Large Geographic Coverage: There are millions of messages posted on social networks every day by users in different locations. Thus, if extracted appropriately, information of interest will have a very large geographic coverage.
- Large Demographic Coverage: In addition, millions of users of different ages, genders, races, or origins, participated in the social media activities every day. The created information can be mined to extract information of interest covering a wide range of demographics.
- Real time: The social media information streams posted in real time allow us to update, track, and monitor events of interest in real time or near real time that surpass the conventional approaches.
- Low Cost: As data is freely accessible and collected from the Internet, the policy makers require less effort and expense compared with the traditional surveying approaches.

Our recent studies showed that mining information from social networks can provide some insights into the activities of marijuana use across the U.S. In this book chapter, we will discuss our techniques used to collect and mine social media streams to extract useful information. The remainder of this book chapter is structured as follows. Section 2 summarizes related work for social network-based approaches for public health applications. In Sect. 3, we present in detail the methodology used in our system, including data collection and data processing methods. Finally, Sect. 4 concludes the chapter.

2 Background and Related Work

2.1 Social Networks

Craigslist
Craigslist is a well-known website for classified advertisements across 700 cities and 70 countries.[1] There are about 80 million classified ads posted each month in different sections devoted to jobs, housing, community, for sale, services, etc. The huge amount of data created by users in Craigslist everyday could suggest the interests or concerns of communities geographically located in different places thanks to the unique web structure of Craigslist, where ads are tagged with locations and of interest of only users living within the vicinity.

---

[1]http://www.craigslist.org/.

Twitter

Twitter is a micro-blogging website that allows users to post messages of 140 characters or less called "tweets".[2] Twitter has become the biggest daily source of news, public opinions, and personal discussions. For example, on the day of the 2016 U.S. presidential election, Twitter had nearly 40 million messages sent by midnight that day [12]. Twitter has 310 million monthly active users, posting hundreds of millions of tweets per day.[3] People on Twitter share, exchange, and discuss any events of their life including various issues relating to their health conditions or health-related behaviors. This phenomena leads to a research area among public health scientists to achieve public health analytic outcomes by harnessing the vast amount of publicly available health-related data.

2.2 Public Health Surveillance via Social Networks

Social networks such as Twitter, Facebook, and Craigslist have quickly become important sources for researchers to track and monitor the public health issues. For example, social media data has been successfully mined and leveraged to empower the near real-time influenza epidemics surveillance. Google Flu Trends track the rate of influenza daily in the U.S. using query logs, several days faster than the Center for Disease Control and Prevention's (CDC) reports [13]. To further improve the performance of influenza detection, researchers in [14] extracted the influenza-related tweets on Twitter then employed machine learning techniques to classify actual messages regarding flu patients. The scheme results in an estimation of at the outbreak and early spread of influenza with high correlation (0.97 correlation) to the official data by the traditional methods. A number of other research enterprises have continued to enhance the influenza prediction accuracy [15, 16]. Notably, [17] introduced a machine learning-based approach fed by the fusion of data from multiple sources including Twitter, Google searchers, hospital visit records, and other existing surveillance systems to provide real-time ("nowcast") estimates of influenza rates in the U.S.

The social media-based surveillance method is also proposed to capture other chronic diseases such as cancer, asthma, toothache, etc. The authors in [18] examined the social network information to get insights into the obesity and diabetes statistics by building a model that maps demographic variables to food names mentioned on Twitter. The system achieved a Pearson correlation of 0.77 with the existing statistics across 50 states in the U.S. Another phenomenon such as cardiac arrest is also monitored from Twitter. The work of [19] collected tweets published in April–May 2011 with keywords cardiac arrest, CPR, AED, resuscitation, heart arrest, sudden death, and defib to learn public knowledge about this disease. They characterized

---

[2]https://twitter.com/.

[3]https://about.twitter.com/company/.

tweets by content, dissemination, and temporal trends. Finally, they used the information retrieved from Twitter to improve resuscitation-related education.

More recently, many researchers have demonstrated the potential for tracking addictive substance use including alcohol and tobacco in the population via social networks. Reference [20] analyzed the content of Twitter posts to detect tobacco-relevant tweets and sentiment toward the new and emerging products like hookah and electronic cigarettes. Several machine learning classifiers such as Naïve Bayes, k-nearest neighbors, and Support Vector Machine were used to detect tobacco-related/not-related tweets as well as positive versus negative sentiment. Another application of social networks includes detecting the activity of quit smoking social network accounts. The authors in [21] collected Twitter users who tweeted the keywords "quit or stop smoking" or "smoking cessation" to detect the evidence of smoking cessation. In addition to tobacco, the researchers found the potential of high exposure of Internet users, especially, children and adolescents to alcohol marketing posts on the social media [22, 23]. The studies suggest that new regulations are needed to impose further restrictions on marketing campaigns regarding addict substances.

2.3 Marijuana in Social Networks

Since the first legalization of recreational marijuana in Colorado in 2012, the public health community started to raise questions about monitoring the marijuana use trend. In an effort to leverage the public content from these sources, the authors in [24] examined the perceptions of marijuana chatters on Twitter to grasp the demographics of the influential Twitter users. Most marijuana-related tweets exhibited a positive attitude from the Twitter members in which the number of pro-marijuana tweets far exceeds that of anti-marijuana tweets (by the factor of 15). Furthermore, more young African–American users tweet the marijuana messages in comparison with the Twitter average. Another approach is using the "visual" social network—Instagram to get some insights about marijuana-related content [25]. The authors acquired 417,561 Instagram marijuana posts with pictures via the related hashtags in November and December 2014, to better understand the new and trendy forms of marijuana consumption together with the marketing of marijuana use.

3 Technical Approaches and Evaluations

3.1 System Architecture

The systematic workflow of our data collecting and processing is illustrated in Fig. 1. We first build a marijuana vocabulary that includes formal and slang words.

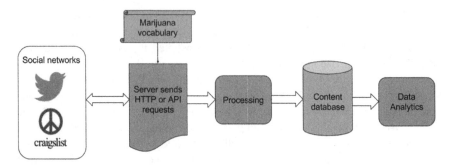

Fig. 1 The workflow of data collection and processing

According to The Online Slang Dictionary,[4] there are at least 180 terms for marijuana, such as pot, weed, 420, stone, etc. The server with Python scripts sends API or HTTP request to the web. While with the Twitter, the script accesses via the REST API, with Craigslist, it calls via the HTTP requests. Depending on the data format, the returned data will be preprocessed before saving into the content database. The preprocessing stage includes removing duplicate and cleaning out the unrelated data. To get the analytic outcomes, we implement several text-mining techniques to extract valuable patterns.

3.2 Revealing Marijuana Use via Craigslist

Data Collection and Processing

Craigslist is a worldwide popular classified advertisements website providing listings in several categories such as jobs, housing, and items wanted.

Figure 2 shows the main page of this website at Chicago. Our research focuses on rental housing posts in the United States and the data collecting process is decomposed into several steps. Firstly, we list all the sites of Craigslist over the entire 50 U.S. states.

In each site, we pick rental house as the desired category to study the marijuana concern. Besides, Craigslist ads are very challenging due to the unstructured ads in which an example is illustrated in Fig. 3.

Therefore, we perform the two following steps before storing significant information in our database:

- Duplicate and Outlier Removal: We also notice that there are many duplicate ads posted on Craigslist despite the no-duplicate policy of Craigslist. So, we remove the duplicate ads which have the same titles including price, location,

---

[4]http://onlineslangdictionary.com.

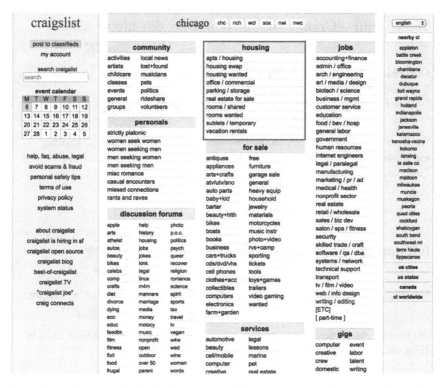

Fig. 2 The main page of Craigslist for the state of Chicago

the number of bedrooms, or those with different titles but the same content will be considered to be duplicated. Our data preprocessing step also filters out all outlier ads with unrealistic prices.

- Extracting Marijuana-Related Ads: Next, we use text mining and semantic analysis algorithm to extract ads with having concerns about the use marijuana. The accuracy of corpus extraction in this step is very important as it determines our data analysis outcome. Interestingly, in our text processing, we found out that the phrases have "420" term such as "420 friendly" or "420 ok" are often used in the ads than the formal phrases have the "marijuana" term itself. However, due to the unstructured texts, we need to filter out "420" unrelated terms. For example, these phrases "#420", "APT 420", "420 bucks per month", "my number is xxx-420-xxxx", etc., appear very often in housing ads but they should not be considered as marijuana-related phrases. Our developed text mining and semantic algorithms have accurately filtered out all of these false positive records.

Table 1 shows some examples of our collected dataset across 50 states in the U. S. After removing the duplicate, outlier, and irrelevant ads, we constructed a dataset of 200,000 rows and 9 columns where each row represents an ad and each column

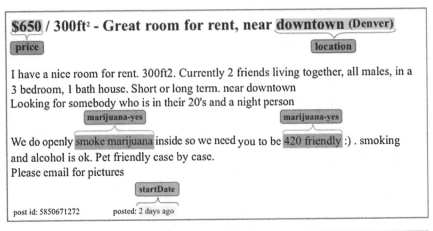

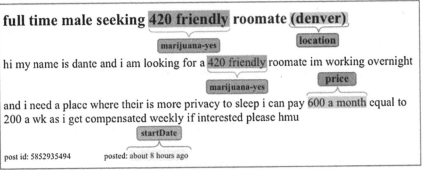

Fig. 3 Examples of annotated ads in Craigslist with information of marijuana use concern, locations, etc.

represents different information extracted from the ad including title of the ad, time listed, state, city, marijuana corpora, rent price, etc. In the dataset, we counted the number of occurrences of each marijuana corpus in different columns. We grouped all marijuana-related corpora with "420" keyword such as "420 is ok", "420 fine", "is 420 allowed" to the field "420 friendly".

Evaluations and Discussions

Our extensive analysis based on the collected data provides some insights into marijuana use and concerns across different states in the U.S. Our data indicated significant differences in marijuana use concerns depending on the legal regulations associated with states and geographic locations. The main findings are summarized in the following subsections.

Table 1 Sample of dataset ("NA" denotes not available data, "0" and "1" are number of counts of the terms in the ad)

Title	State	Location	Price	tratDat	Bedroom	"420 friendly"	"Marijuana"	"Cannabis"
Hoover House 4 bedroom/2.5 bath home	CO	Denver	1600	2016-1	4br	1	0	0
Wow-cute, clean cottage-gated resort	OR	Portland	75	2016-1	NA	0	1	0
Share a big room near downtown	CO	Denver	1250	2016-1	1br	1	0	0
$1200/2br—950 ft^2—Awesome 2 bedroom 1 bath	AK	Anchorage	1200	2016-1	2br	1	0	0
Awesome 2 bd, 1 bath! Large yard w/storage!	AK	Anchorage	1200	2016-1	2br	1	1	0
In transition? Flexible lease available	OR	Portland	NA	2016-1	NA	0	0	1

Marijuana-Related Terms

In our data analysis, we found out that "marijuana" term is not the most often used term to describe marijuana-related concerns (e.g., allowed or not allowed use of marijuana). This is a surprising result at first as based on the existing studies we expected "marijuana"-related keywords should be the most often used term. By further carefully examining all marijuana-related terms, both formal and slang ones in the "housing" category, surprisingly, we found that "420" term (e.g., "420 friendly") is most often used in the rental ads to indicate marijuana use concerns, instead of "marijuana"-related keywords. More specifically, we found out that the "420" term used the most in two subcategories "room & shares" and "room/share wanted", appear more than ten times as the "marijuana"-related keywords as shown in Table 2 and about four times more than total of all other marijuana-related keywords used. This finding is very interesting as it suggests a new term to indicate "marijuana" term when conducting text mining.

Our result is a great complement to the existing studies on marijuana-related aspects in online platforms such as [24, 26]. Those studies skip very important "420" marijuana-related keywords when investigating marijuana-related content on Twitter.

The Division of Rental World in Marijuana-Related Ads

Our study further revealed the difference of keyword usages in describing marijuana concerns between organizations and private lessors. Based on our collected data, we compared the number of rental ads with and without marijuana-related terms from subcategories "office & commercial" in which listings are from rental companies. In this analysis, we only focused on four marijuana-legalizing states including Colorado, Washington, Oregon, and Alaska. The data indicates that rental companies tend to use formal keywords such as "marijuana" or "cannabis" while the private parties used "420"-related keywords more often as indicated in Table 2. Table 3 shows the total number of posts containing term "marijuana", "cannabis", and "420"-related term in four states within one month.

Table 2 Summary of marijuana-related terms in subcategories of "housing" in the state of Colorado

Marijuana-related terms summary					
Category	T1	T2	T3	T4	T5
Rooms & shares	1012	387	26	38	149
Room/share wanted	418	46	35	55	19
Apts/housing for rent	148	340	128	41	91
Sublets & temporary	108	42	11	17	39
Total	1686	591	200	151	298

T1 = "420 friendly", T2 = "marijuana", T3 = "mmj", T4 = "cannabis", and T5 = "pot"

Table 3 Summary of marijuana-related terms in subcategory "office & commercial"

States	Office & commercial subcategory		
	"Marijuana"	"Cannabis"	"420 friendly"
Colorado	223	68	14
Washington	181	29	13
Oregon	497	303	7
Alaska	23	25	2

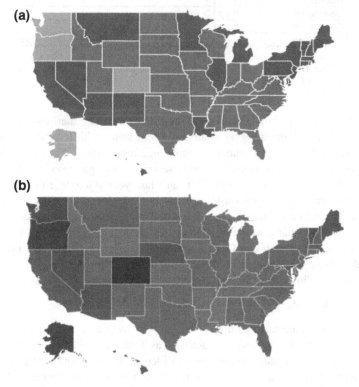

Fig. 4 Comparison of **a** state marijuana laws map and **b** geographical distribution of marijuana-related corpora ads in Craigslist (number of listings per population)

Comparing to the Marijuana State Laws Map and Google Marijuana Keyword Search.

To validate and verify our data collected on Craigslist about marijuana use, we linked the ads to their geographic locations and used colored map to indicate the number of related keywords used across 50 states in the U.S. Figure 4 displays the marijuana state laws map as of May 2016[5] (Fig. 4a) and our marijuana-related

---

[5]http://www.governing.com/gov-data/state-marijuana-laws-map-medical-recreational.html.

(a)

	Google 5Y	Google 3Y	Google 1Y	Craig. Norm.
Google 5Y	1			
Google 3Y	0.98	1		
Google 1Y	0.89	0.93	1	
Craig. Norm.	0.62	0.59	0.33	1

(b)

	Google 5Y	Google 3Y	Google 1Y	Craig. Norm.
Google 5Y	1			
Google 3Y	0.99	1		
Google 1Y	0.99	0.97	1	
Craig. Norm.	0.71	0.72	0.66	1

Fig. 5 Correlation table of Google Marijuana keyword search versus Marijuana-related corpora ads in Craigslist **a** all states; **b** top 10 states

corpora ads extracted from Craigslist (Fig. 4b). In the state marijuana laws map, light green, dark green, and gray colors represent states with legalizing marijuana for recreation, for medical, and not legalizing, respectively. Figure 5a, b show correlation tables of marijuana keyword search in Google over last five years (Google 5Y), three years (Google 3Y), and last year (Google 1Y) versus state population-normalized marijuana-related ads in Craigslist of the 50 states and top 10 states. The data collected in Craigslist with "marijuana"-related ads are strongly correlated with the states where marijuana uses are legal in some forms in both the state marijuana laws map and Google search. This is expected, as marijuana uses are legal in those states; thus, lessors more often use marijuana-related corpora (e.g., allowed or not allowed) in their ads to attract more lessees.

Marijuana Black Market: The Hidden World Revealed

Interestingly, our data revealed that the terms "420"-related words which have been used very often in the ads in some states such as Texas, Florida, or Nevada in Fig. 6 where the use of marijuana in any form is illegal. Based on the federal laws and state marijuana laws map, we expected that less or no ads with concerns about the use of marijuana would be posted in those states because, obviously, no one in those areas is allowed to use marijuana in any forms. Surprisingly, our data indicated a contrary observation. A significant number of rental ads included marijuana-related keywords in their ads have been posted in these areas. For example, Florida has more than 900 ads posted with marijuana-related keywords. From the business and public health aspects, these ads suggest some level of actual marijuana use in those communities; thus, the ads have been crafted with those keywords to attract more lessees in these areas. In other words, the evidence from the collected data can be interpreted as there exists some level of illegal marijuana use in those states and the findings shed some light on those aspects that authorities and public health agencies should develop appropriate policy and regulation to restrain the reality of the marijuana use.

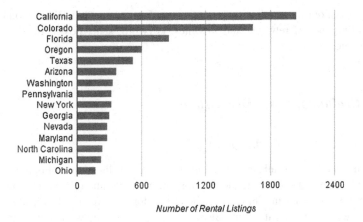

Fig. 6 Frequencies of "420 friendly" corpora in the "housing" category

3.3 Characterizing Marijuana Activities via Tweets

Data Collections and Processing

Twitter provides developers several APIs to create tweets, read user profile, follower data, in which the Search API is useful in monitoring and searching tweets in real time. Therefore, we have conducted experiments on Twitter data during November 2016, collected and processed more than 300,000 marijuana-related tweets in the English language. Next, the server component, written in Python, interacts with the Twitter Search API to collect data from Twitter data source. While the Twitter Search API usually serves up to date Tweets, our system allows us to bypass this limitation of time constraints by basically replicating the way the Twitter Search engine works on browsers. Using marijuana-related terms stored in Vocabulary component, the server calls the API by the command: "https://twitter. com/i/search/timeline?f=realtime" with following parameters:

- **q**: a query text in which searched tweets will contain. It is a word and phrase relating to marijuana, pre-stored in our vocabulary.
- **since**: the lower bound of the posting date of searched tweets.
- **until**: the upper bound of the posting date of searched tweets.
- **lang**: the language of searched tweets.

This API retrieves a list of matched tweets in the form of an HTML string. Finally, the server extracts useful data from HTML string and save them to our tweet database component. The resulting tweets are stored in a NoSQL tweet database which includes $316,191$ documents relating to marijuana. Each document represents a tweet with 15 different fields extracted from the JSON object resulted from our data collection process, including username, URL, external links, text, the number of retweets and favorites, keyword, state, posted time, types of devices, etc.

3.4 Evaluations and Discussions

Marijuana Unigram and Bigram Clouds

Unigrams and bigrams allow generating cloud tags for illustration of popular terms. Figure 7a shows the most frequent terms among unigrams (after removing some most common terms in English). Generally, "dope", "weed", "pot", and "marijuana" are some highlight words. Besides those four favorite words, there are many action words associated with marijuana consumption such as "smoke", "smoking", "buy", "like", "love", and "smell". Interestingly, data extracted from our text-mining algorithm indicated that there were many terms with provocative meaning such as "ass", "bitch", "shit", or "dam" are usually used in marijuana tweets. In addition, our data also shows a strong correlation between a number of tweets and some geographical locations, which appeared have substantial activities related to cannabis. For example, Colorado, which has firstly legalized using marijuana for adult 21 years of age or older, is mentioned most. This suggests that legalization of marijuana in many areas has sparked a controversy, including positive and negative opinions.

Figure 7b reveals more-detailed information of marijuana use via the bigram cloud. Apparently, this type of cloud clearly shows many marijuana-related vocabularies such as legal, melting, dope, super, crock, etc. Also, the frequency of pair words which is related to legalization is very popular. It may reflect the event of state legalization votes during November. The frequency of "medical marijuana"

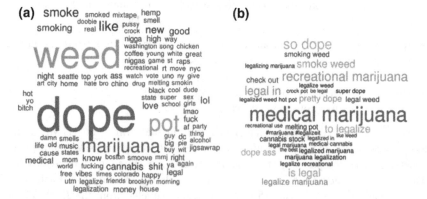

Fig. 7 Unigram cloud (**a**) and Bigram cloud (**b**) of marijuana-related tweets collected during November 2016

Table 4 Top 20 users posted marijuana-related tweets with external links

User	Number of links	Place
Potnetworkcom	1638	Denver, Co
eatin_n_streets	1582	Denver, Co
DenverCP	764	Denver, Co
DiegoPellicer	654	Seattle, WA
MME_MESA	424	Mesa, AZ
ermphd	410	Austin, TX
OG_Chino	397	Los Angeles, CA
ABG_Marketplace	343	Kansas City, MO
WeedFeed	271	Chicago, IL
Boston_CP	270	Boston, MA
SLM420LOVE	269	California, CA
CoCannabisCo	266	Oregon, OR
SpeakEasy_SEVL	252	Colorado Springs, CO
Chance_Takers	243	Atlanta, GA
greco_james	238	Phoenix, AZ
Diabetes_Newzz	236	New York, NY
PhoenixCP	233	Phoenix, AZ
420digitalweb	224	Denver, Co
Cannabis_Card	212	San Diego, LA
StartupCannabis	206	New York, NY

indicates that more and more users want to promote the benefit of using marijuana for medical purposes.

Identifying Users' Attitudes via Tweets

Our data indicates that we can actually distinguish users' attitudes toward cannabis use via the number of outer links in their tweets. Outer links or external links are identified, based on the total number of URLs in the tweet metadata including full URLs and shortened URLs. Particularly, more than 300,000 tweets in our database, there are total 158,814 tweets without outer links and 157,377 tweets with outer links. Table 4 shows top 20 users who had outer links in their tweets. Our data analysis reveals that most of these users (17/20) were from states where the use of marijuana for medical purpose or recreational use is legal (e.g., Colorado, Washington, Illinois, Massachusetts, California, and New York). For example, top three users with most tweets containing external links, unsurprisingly, come from Denver, Colorado—one of the first states where marijuana is legal for both medical and recreational purpose. More specifically, we find out that most of these users are likely to be news and magazine organizations such as Potnetworkcom, DenverCP, PhoenixCP, Boston_CP, WeedFeed, and MME_MESA. For example, user Potnetworkcom with 1638 tweets has a website http://potnetwork.com/—that

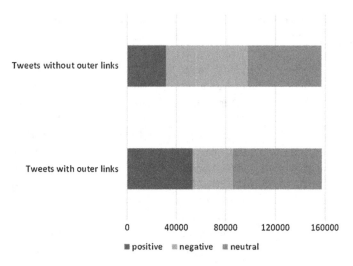

Fig. 8 Sentiment analysis of 158,814 tweets without outer links and 157,377 tweets with outer links: Tweets without outer links seem to be more negative than ones with outer links

publishes all things about Marijuana and entertains other users "with up to date information about marijuana pop culture" or DenverPC belongs to website http:// toplocalnow.com/ that tweets breaking news and weather updates from Denver and many other cities. Our data reveals that many organizations, which provide services and products associated with marijuana, tend to utilize Twitter to promote their products and generate publicity.

We use a tweet sentiment analysis tool by Mashape[6] to estimate the Twitter user attitude toward Cannabis. The tool works by examining individual words and short sequences of words (*n*-grams) and comparing them with a probability model. We analyze two sets: the tweets with outer links and tweets without outer links for evaluation. In Fig. 8, we present information about the proportion of the sentiment. Overall, for the set of tweets with URLs, the percentage of positive tweets is higher than the negative tweets. For the set of tweets without URLs, however, the percentage of positive tweets is much lower. Considering the group of positive tweets, the proportion of the positive tweet with external links is 62%, compared with 32% of tweets without external links. This implies that many users who attach external links to some websites try to deliver the information about the benefits of marijuana, such as for medical and experiments. They might want other people to perceive the advantages of marijuana. Users, who do not attach URLs in their tweets, can be individual marijuana smokers. However, because of many offensive terms (e.g., "bitch", or alike words) included in their tweets, they are identified as having negative sentiments toward marijuana.

---

[6]https://www.mashape.com/.

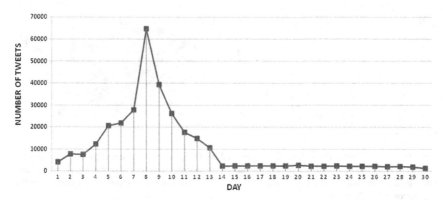

Fig. 9 Daily distribution of the number of tweets relating to marijuana in November 2016: there is an exponential increase in the number of marijuana-related tweets during the week of the US presidential election and legalization votes in some more states

Temporal and Spatial Distribution of Tweets

The volume of marijuana-related discussions is largely driven by political events. Figure 9 shows the daily distribution of the number of tweets relating to marijuana in November 2016. Clearly, in the first week of the month, the number of tweets increased at an exponential rate and reached a peak on November 8. The tweets express the user's emotion and opinion about the marijuana policy reforms. For example, on November 9 four more states (California, Nevada, Maine, and Massachusetts in addition to Colorado, Washington, Alaska, Oregon, and Washington DC) voted for legal marijuana consumption of both recreational and medical purpose [27]. Another important reason is that the same period, the outcome of US presidential election was decided and the elected president has shown support for using cannabis for medical purpose and is likely to encourage the federal government to allow more states to vote on legalizing recreational marijuana [28].

It is interesting to estimate the tweet frequency during the regular weeks, i.e., without special effects of presidential elections or marijuana legalization events. We, therefore, consider the time from November 15 to 31.

The research presented at [29] proves there are more tweets about alcohol during the weekend. This is also true for marijuana. Figure 10a presents a daily distribution of marijuana-related tweets in regular weeks, i.e., excluding the abnormal weeks of U.S. Election Day 2016 and cannabis legalization election days. We observe a clear trend that there is a significant uptick in the number of tweets at the weekend as compared to weekdays. We make a prediction that at the weekend, users tend to have more spare time to enjoy recreational activities. Also, Twitter accounts of celebrities, the media or businesses might exploit the value of weekend tweeting to post more tweets since their audiences have more time to consume and share content.

By the end of November 2016, there are eight states including California, Nevada, Maine, and Massachusetts, Colorado, Washington, Alaska, and Oregon,

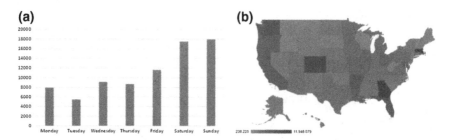

Fig. 10 **a** Daily distribution of marijuana-related tweets in a week during November 2016—the average for the whole month excluding the day of presidential election and marijuana legalization vote; **b** the state map of the marijuana-related tweet frequencies (the number of tweets over the population of each state)

and Washington DC which have been legalized to use marijuana for both recreational and medical purpose.[7] Our spatial graph in Fig. 10b shows that there are more tweets from those eight states, thus matching with the marijuana state law map in 2016. The number of tweets, however, is also quite high in some states such as Georgia. Based on the federal laws and state marijuana laws map, we expect that fewer marijuana-related tweets in this state because this area only allows for limited medical purposes. Surprisingly, our data indicated a contrary observation. This can be interpreted, as there is some level of marijuana use beyond the medical purposes. Further study on such issues is considered as our future work.

It is known that 82% of active users are on mobile phones.[8] This raises us a question on the device types of marijuana tweeting users. Within more than 91,000 users we process, about 67% use mobile phones (51% for iPhone and 16% for Android phones) via the Twitter mobile application to post their tweets (Fig. 11).

There are about 8695 users who use Internet browsers such as Chrome, Firefox, and Safari that are in the group of Twitter Web Client. Importantly, many users (remaining 23.5%) employ third-party services to publish their marijuana-related tweets. Two such popular services are IFTTT and TweetDeck. IFTTT, an abbreviation of "If This Then That", is a web-based service that allows users to tweet automatically based on schedules or some particular events. Similarly, TweetDeck is a Twitter tool for real-time tracking, organizing, and engagement that helps users to reach their audiences by automatic postings. Thus, there is an unusually less number of users using mobile devices when comparing to the average number of 82%. Our observed data can explain that in the marijuana-related tweets, many users are employing automated posting services to promote their products or implementing marketing strategies.

---

[7]http://www.governing.com/gov-data/state-marijuana-laws-map-medical-recreational.html.
[8]https://about.twitter.com/company.

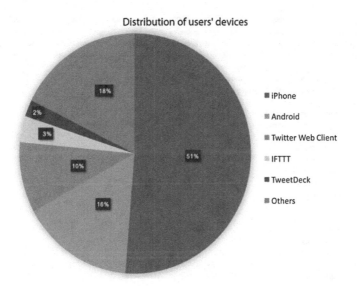

Distribution of users' devices

- iPhone
- Android
- Twitter Web Client
- IFTTT
- TweetDeck
- Others

Fig. 11 The proportion of devices of the users who post marijuana-related tweets on Twitter

Marijuana-related Hashtags

Topics in Tweeter are categorized based on hashtags, labeling words or phrases preceded by a pound sign (#). By using hashtags, Twitter's users can express their tweet's content, and thus, specific subjects of discussions among users can be found more quickly.

Figure 12 illustrates most common hashtags among marijuana-related discussions. Unsurprisingly, #marijuana #cannabis #dope and #weed are the most ubiquitous terms. Besides, other marijuana-related hashtags are also frequently used such as #pot, #kush, #mmj, #hemp, #cbd, and #thc. Two terms #cbd and #thc, respectively, refer to Cannabidiol and Tetrahydrocannabinol, two main ingredients in the marijuana plant. #mmj means "marijuana".

We also notice that some political hashtags frequently appear such as #legalizeit, #electionnight, #electionnday, #vote, and #YESon. #YESon means "Yes on", a typical phrase used by Twitter users in the election campaigns. There might be a variety of reasons for this circumstance. Firstly, our dataset is collected during November 2016. During this time, nine states were voting for marijuana legalization, including Florida, Massachusetts, North Dakota, Maine, Arkansas, Montana, Arizona, Nevada, and California. On November 8, California, Nevada, Maine, and Massachusetts all voted for legalized use, sale, and consumption of recreational marijuana. Secondly, the appearance of political hashtags #electionnight, #electionnday, and #vote reflects US presidential election event happening at the same time. It is clear that the presidential candidates' attitudes and the new government's policy toward the state marijuana legalization trend will dramatically affect every

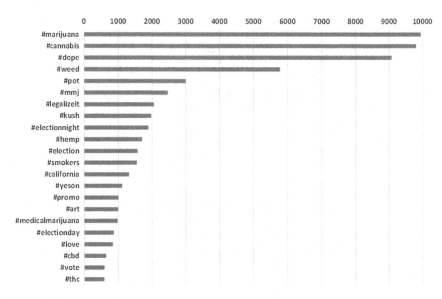

Fig. 12 Top 20 hashtags in marijuana-related tweets: #marijuana, #cannabis, #dope, and #weed are most common hashtags

marijuana business and individual who consumes marijuana, just provoking a lot of discussions on this topic.

4 Conclusion

This book chapter describes some preliminary results of a new research trend by using social media to track and monitor the perception and consumption of the emerging addictive substances such as marijuana. We conducted our collecting and mining techniques for cannabis-related content from two well-known social network websites: Craigslist and Twitter. Firstly, we developed lightweight text-mining algorithms to extract marijuana-related corpus from unstructured ads in Craigslist to reveal the geographic distributions of marijuana use. Our result indicates a strong correlation of ads with marijuana use concerns with the state marijuana laws map and Google marijuana keyword search in states where the marijuana use is legal. Interestingly, our data also reveals some strong concerns about marijuana use in other states, where possession of marijuana in any form is illegal. Second, we also performed some statistical data analysis on marijuana content from Twitter during November 2016. The study exhibited some interesting patterns including the frequencies of the Unigrams and Bigram of marijuana tweets. The opinion of state marijuana legalization votes and the US presidential election, some levels of association between users who tweet with and without external links, the distribution of user devices, the frequencies of posts within a week, and the differences between the way and purpose of the individual users and the organizational users. Those findings would suggest some valuable patterns which could be used as a marijuana surveillance approach for federal authorities and public health agencies in developing policy and regulations. More importantly, the results promise a forward step toward online marijuana surveillance capable of providing a larger geographic–demographic coverage with low cost and time efficiency.

References

1. Abuse, S.: Mental Health Services Administration (2014) Results from the 2013 national survey on drug use and health (2014)
2. Volkow, N.D., Baler, R.D., Compton, W.M., Weiss, S.R.: Adverse health effects of marijuana use. N. Engl. J. Med. **370**(23), 2219–2227 (2014)
3. Hall, W., Degenhardt, L.: The adverse health effects of chronic cannabis use. Drug Testing Anal **6**(1–2), 39–45 (2014)
4. Greydanus, D.E., Hawver, E.K., Greydanus, M.M.: 8 marijuana: current concepts and conundrums. In: Substance Abuse in Adolescents and Young Adults: A Manual for Pediatric and Primary Care Clinicians (2013)
5. Blanco, C., Hasin, D.S., Wall, M.M., Flórez-Salamanca, L., Hoertel, N., Wang, S., Kerridge, B.T., Olfson, M.: Cannabis use and risk of psychiatric disorders: prospective evidence from a US national longitudinal study. JAMA Psychiatry **73**(4), 388–395 (2016)
6. Batalla, A., Bhattachayyria, S., Yucel, M., Fusar-Poli, P., Crippa, J.A., Nogué, S., Torrens, M., Pujol, J., Farré, M., Martín-Santos, R.: Structural and functional imaging studies in chronic cannabis users: a systematic review of adolescent and adult findings. Euro Psychiatry **28**, 1 (2013)
7. Hartman, R.L., Huestis, M.A.: Cannabis effects on driving skills. Clin. Chem. **59**(3), 478–492 (2013)
8. Dredze, M.: How social media will change public health. IEEE Intell. Syst. **27**(4), 81–84 (2012)
9. Paul, M., Dredze, M., Broniatowski, D., Generous, N.: Worldwide influenza surveillance through twitter. In: Shaban-Nejad, A., Buckeridge, D.L., Brownstein, J.S. (eds.) Proceedings of AAAI Workshop on the World Wide Web and Public Health Intelligence (2015)
10. Macleod, J., Oakes, R., Copello, A., Crome, I., Egger, M., Hickman, M., Oppenkowski, T., Stokes-Lampard, H., Smith, G.D.: Psychological and social sequelae of cannabis and other illicit drug use by young people: a systematic review of longitudinal, general population studies. The Lancet **363**(9421), 1579–1588 (2004)
11. Azofeifa, A., Mattson, M.E., Schauer, G., McAfee, T., Grant, A., Lyerla, R.: National estimates of marijuana use and related indicators—national survey on drug use and health, United States, 2002-2014. MMWR. Surveill Summ, 1–25 (2016)
12. Isaac, M., Ember, S.: For election day influence, twitter ruled social media (2016)
13. Carneiro, H.A., Mylonakis, E.: Google trends: a web-based tool for real-time surveillance of disease outbreaks. Clin. Infect. Dis. 1557–1564 (2009)
14. Aramaki, E., Maskawa, S., Morita, M.: Twitter catches the flu: detecting influenza epidemics using Twitter. In: Proceedings of the Conference on Empirical Methods in Natural Language Processing (2011)
15. Lamb, M., Paul, J., Dredze, M.: Separating fact from fear: tracking flu infections on Twitter. In: HLT-NAACL (2013)

16. Smith, M., Broniatowski, D.A., Paul, M.J., Dredze, M.: Towards real-time measurement of public epidemic awareness: monitoring influenza awareness through twitter (2015)
17. Santillana, M., Nguyen, A.T., Dredze, M., Paul, M.J., Nsoesie, E.O., Brownstein, J.S.: Combining search, social media, and traditional data sources to improve influenza surveillance. PLoS Comput. Biol. 11(10), e1004513 (2015)
18. Abbar, S., Mejova, Y., Weber, I.: You tweet what you eat: studying food consumption through twitter. In: Proceedings of the 33rd Annual ACM Conference on Human Factors in Computing Systems (2015)
19. Bosley, J.C., Zhao, N.W., Hill, S., Shofer, F.S., Asch, D.A., Becker, L.B., Merchant, R.M.: Decoding twitter: surveillance and trends for cardiac arrest and resuscitation communication. Resuscitation 84(2), 206–212 (2013)
20. Myslín, M., Zhu, S.-H., Chapman, W., Conway, M.: Using twitter to examine smoking behavior and perceptions of emerging tobacco products. J. Med. Internet Res. 15(8), e174 (2013)
21. Prochaska, J.J., Pechmann, C., Kim, R., Leonhardt, J.M.: Twitter = quitter? An analysis of Twitter quit smoking social networks. Tobacco Control 21(4), 447–449 (2012)
22. Nicholls, J.: Everyday, everywhere: alcohol marketing and social media—current trends. Alcohol. Alcohol. 47(4), 486–493 (2012)
23. Winpenny, E.M., Marteau, T.M., Nolte, E.: Exposure of children and adolescents to alcohol marketing on social media websites. Alcohol. Alcohol. 49(2), 154–159 (2014)
24. Cavazos-Rehg, P.A., Krauss, M., Fisher, S.L., Salyer, P., Grucza, R.A., Bierut, L.J.: Twitter chatter about marijuana. J. Adolesc. Health 56(2), 139–145 (2015)
25. Cavazos-Rehg, P.A., Krauss, M.J., Sowles, S.J., Bierut, L.J.: Marijuana-related posts on Instagram. Prev. Sci. 17(6), 710–720 (2016)
26. Daniulaityte, R., Nahhas, R.W., Wijeratne, S., Carlson, R.G., Lamy, F.R., Martins, S.S., Boyer, E.W., Smith, G.A., Sheth, A.: "Time for dabs": analyzing Twitter data on marijuana concentrates across the U.S. Drug Alcohol Depend. 155, 307–311 (2015)
27. Gilbert, B.: 4 states just voted to make marijuana completely legal—here's what we know (2016)
28. Berke, J.: Here's where Donald Trump and Hillary Clinton stand on marijuana legalization (2016)
29. Kypri, K., Davie, G., McElduff, P., Connor, J., Langley, J., Wang, H., Hovy, E., Dredze, M.: Effects of lowering the minimum alcohol purchasing age on weekend assaults resulting in hospitalization in New Zealand. Am. J. Public Health 104(8), 1396–1401 (2014)

Online Public Health Intelligence: Ethical Considerations at the Big Data Era

Hiroshi Mamiya, Arash Shaban-Nejad and David L. Buckeridge

Abstract Often times terms such as Big Data, increasing digital footprints in the Internet accompanied with advancing analytical techniques, represent a major opportunity to improve public health surveillance and delivery of interventions. However, early adaption of Big Data in other fields revealed ethical challenges that could undermine privacy and autonomy of individuals and cause stigmatization. This chapter aims to identify the benefits and risks associated with the public health application of Big Data through ethical lenses. In doing so, it highlights the need for ethical discussion and framework towards an effective utilization of technologies. We then discuss key strategies to mitigate potentially harmful aspects of Big Data to facilitate its safe and effective implementation.

Keywords Public health ethics · Privacy · Public health surveillance · Public health intervention · Big Data health analytics · Online social media

1 Introduction

Primary objectives of public health agencies are to protect and promote the health of citizens through population-based strategies [1]. Public health actions include legal measures such as mandated use of seatbelt and motorcycle helmets, taxation

H. Mamiya (✉) · D.L. Buckeridge
Department of Epidemiology and Biostatistics and Occupational Health, McGill University, Montreal, QC, Canada
e-mail: hiroshimamiya@gmail.com

D.L. Buckeridge
e-mail: david.buckeridge@mcgill.ca

A. Shaban-Nejad
Department of Pediatrics, Oak-Ridge National Laboratories (UTHSC-ORNL)
Center for Biomedical Informatics, University of Tennessee Health Science Center, Memphis, TN, USA
e-mail: ashabann@uthsc.edu

© Springer International Publishing AG 2017   129
A. Shaban-Nejad et al. (eds.), *Public Health Intelligence and the Internet*,
Lecture Notes in Social Networks, https://doi.org/10.1007/978-3-319-68604-2_8

of unhealthy food and mandatory reporting, testing and treatment of serious communicable diseases. Voluntary measures include preventive programs such as vaccination, educational campaigns for promoting healthy lifestyle, and nutrition supplementation to economically disadvantaged populations. Because health and health-related behaviors of populations can be highly influenced by environmental factors such as air pollution, green space, retail food environment, and hygiene, public health agencies are also responsible for improving the living environment [2]. An equally important role of public health is the surveillance of population health status, which encompasses spatiotemporal distribution of disease outcomes, behavioral risk factors, and physical and social environment affecting health. As a backbone of public health activities, surveillance provides critical insights in population health status to guide the development, management, and evaluation of interventions. As well, surveillance has a critical role in identifying of health needs among disadvantaged populations, thereby assisting the development of equitable health interventions.

The role of public health agencies considerably expanded from solely tracking and controlling of communicable diseases that were the primary cause of mortality up to the early twentieth century [3]. Noncommunicable diseases such as cancer, cardiovascular diseases, and diabetes, are now responsible for the majority of global death and disability [4], which placed increasing importance on the monitoring and preventive interventions for lifestyle risk factors such as diet, physical activities, and tobacco use. Socioeconomic and demographic inequality in health remains an important public health problem requiring the development and evaluation of equitable intervention reaching to underprivileged individuals. Other critical public health mandates include prevention and surveillance of injuries, assessment of healthcare performance, improvement of maternal and infant health, and disaster response. Furthermore, health of public is threatened by the resurgence of vaccine-preventable diseases [5, 6] and constantly emerging infectious diseases with significant national and global health consequence, including Severe Acute Respiratory Syndrome (SARS), West Nile Virus, the 2009 pandemic H1N1 influenza, and more recently the epidemic of Ebola hemorrhagic fever in the West Africa [7]. Ever-growing complexity and breadth of public health tasks call for innovative answers strengthening capacity of health agencies.

1.1 Ethical Challenges in Public Health Practice

Although individual liberties such as the right to privacy and autonomy represent a fundamental importance in our society, public health agency's obligation to maximize community good and societal well-being inevitably conflicts with these values [8]. As an example, mandatory reporting and disclosure of personal information [9] in the name-based control of human immunodeficiency virus (HIV) imposed privacy threats and stigmatization among infected and heterosexual men [10, 11], whereas the control of tuberculosis (TB) often resulted in the use of police power to enforce isolation and detainment of diseased individuals and their contacts.

In addition, health promotion programs (e.g., promotion of healthy diet and physical exercise) can lead to victim blaming and stereotyping towards individuals with stigmatizing conditions such as obesity, treating the failure to comply healthy lifestyle as a matter of personal responsibility [12]. Policy intervention is invariably challenged by individualism and libertarian advocates [13], as exemplified by the opposing arguments against motor vehicle helmet law claiming excessive state's police power and paternalism acted upon the liberty of the riders and discrimination in classifying them as a high-risk class, despite overwhelmingly positive evidence for the use of motor vehicle helmet in preventing death [14].

As for disease surveillance, public health agencies are exempted from routine ethics review and obtaining informed consent from patients to access to personally identifiable information that are collected for public and nonpublic health purposes, such as patient care and medical billing [9, 11, 15]. Although the exemption is necessary in a setting where immediate access to personal data and subsequent actions are paramount as in the control of certain communicable diseases such amendment was also extended to the monitoring of noncommunicable diseases, often sparking dispute in the limit of data access [16]. Breach of patient health information is a critical confidentiality problem considering the amount of personal data analysts, yet such incidence is surprisingly common among local health agencies [17, 18].

Taken together, public health intervention and practice are subject to a considerable moral challenge and longstanding dispute in seeking a trade-off between preservation of individual's liberties and collective benefits of the population.

1.2 Big Data and Web 2.0 Technologies

The web and mobile applications supported by the Web 2.0 technologies led to unprecedented growth of personal information and communication footprints available in the Internet. The technologies and devices that surround modern lives continuously capture digital traces of daily activities including financial, environmental, and social interactions. The advances in "Big Data" [19] research has created a unique opportunity to process these networks of heterogeneous data to generate explanatory and predictive models [20], leading to field applications in commercial and political sectors to generate insights into and influence voter and consumer behaviors [21]. As an example, online browsing records are routinely used to monitor credit card fraud, develop individually targeted marketing, and create customer segmentation [21–23].

Big Data can be loosely explained by the following three dimensions: (*i*) Volume that explains how large is the datasets; (*ii*) Velocity that indicates how fast these large datasets are processed, and (*iii*) Variety, which refers to how different are these datasets in sources and formats [24]. Although defining Web 2.0

requires technical discussion [25], in the context of public health application, we characterize the term as a group of technologies allowing web applications/services to: (*a*) provide capabilities to upload and share contents by users; (*b*) harness collective intelligence extracted from the user contributed data; (*c*) provide dynamic and tailored contents matched to user's profile or needs; and (*d*) the use web as platform, thus runs in wide range of devices. Some examples of Web 2.0 applications/services are search engines, blogs, multimedia sharing websites (e.g., YouTube), social networking services (SNS), and business review websites (e.g., Yelp).

Although the application of Big Data and Web 2.0 applications/services in public health activities is largely in its infancy, their potential in enhancing the capacity of surveillance and intervention led to a raised enthusiasm [26–30]. Shadowed by the excitement, however, ethical consequences of implementing these technologies received inadequate attention to date [31, 32]. As the earlier adoption in commercial sector revealed their privacy harming aspects and resulting public concerns towards the indiscriminate use of personal data by industries [21, 33], it is imperative to address the potential benefits on health of public and risks to individuals liberties of Big Data and Web 2.0 applications/technologies. Following section describes their opportunities of in advancing the science and practice of public health, followed by potential harms upon application to public health surveillance and intervention from the ethical perspective. Finally, we provide strategies to mitigate the risks in a hope to provide an initial step towards the development of legal safeguards and guidelines.

2 Opportunities of Big Data and Web 2.0 Technologies

The digital stream of personal, environmental, and social attributes can be gathered and analyzed at a large scale, whereas web applications and mobile devices provide means to reach a large number of individuals at relatively low cost [34].

The transformative features of digital/mobile and participatory technology include ability to assess citizen sentiment and deliver individually tailored (targeted) message at low cost [35], peer support for proactive and positive health-related behaviors among online community [36], timely access to citizen report at global scale through "crowdsourcing" [37, 38], and improved outreach to young and socioeconomically deprived individuals [39, 40]. In addition, the widespread use of digital devices (e.g., mobile phones) provides effective communication channel for reporting disease outbreaks by citizen sentinel network in low-resource settings [41]. In effect, participatory surveillance offers a potential to create a mutual collaboration between public health agencies and citizen sentinel who submits local information and in return receives relevant information to their context. This is contrary to the current use of online data by commercial industries, where the users' data is routinely sold and/or analyzed by service providers (although aggregated or anonymized), and the profit from inferred/discovered knowledge is not shared with the Internet users, while the users suffer from privacy intrusion [23].

From the perspective of social justice, an equally important blessing of the mobile communication technology is their outreach to population subgroups that were previously unreceptive to or unreachable by traditional communication channels, for whom health disparity often exists [42, 43]. Finally, given the ongoing shift of citizen communication and information seeking to the digital environments [40], surveillance of online information and communication environment is likely to be an essential task to identify emerging public health challenges such as online advertisement of unhealthy products.

2.1 User Engagement and Empowerment

Traditional public health communication has been largely unidirectional and uniform. Health promotion, risk communication, and educational messages were typically disseminated through traditional media (e.g., television, radio, and printed media) without reflection of the individual context and needs [44]. The user centrality of the Web 2.0 applications/services has a potential to increase citizen engagement with public health messages through personalized and tailored contents [39, 44, 45]. Tailoring is particularly suited to convey clear and relevant information to those who are lacking sufficient health and technology literacy. In addition, interactive and synchronous nature of these technologies can promote bidirectional communications between public health organizations and users, potentially allowing health agencies to respond to user inquiries, share ideas, and encourage user-generated health contents [39] as well as facilitating peer supports and sharing of experience within the communities.

Furthermore, collaborative characteristic of the Internet can mitigate the effect of victim blaming due to stereotyping and labeling by media [46] by providing an environment for peer-supporting communities that can empower socially underprivileged individuals with stigmatized health conditions, such as obesity and HIV [47, 48]. As well, the openness of the Internet provides an opportunity for activism and resistance against "culture of stigma" or public ridicule towards these individuals [47, 49, 50].

2.2 Population Reach

In the United States, the digital divide in terms of access to the Internet is gradually closing across socioeconomic and demographic groups. In 2015, 74% of low-income individuals reported Internet usage, a 40% increase from 2000, and the gap in Internet adoption between high- and low-income groups shrunk from 47% in 2000 to 23% in 2015 [51]. Turning to education, 64% those without high school diploma used the Internet in 2015, relative to 19% in 2000, narrowing the gap from 59% in 2000 to 29% in 2015 [51]. Across age groups, Internet usage showed the steepest increase among seniors, climbing from 14% in 2000 to 58% in 2015. Driving this change is the widespread use of smartphones, which are owned by nearly two-thirds of adults in 2015 in developed nations, and undergoing rapid uptake in developing nations [52, 53]. In addition, the socioeconomic difference in the use of SNS appears to be absent in the U.S. [54], which suggests the equitable quality of health promotion through this channel.

Combined with the anonymity of the Internet, the wide population outreach is particularly effective in addressing sensitive and stigmatized topics among hard-to-reach individuals, such as men who have sex with men, older adolescents and young adults, and those affected by mental illness [40, 55]. As an example, the Internet has become a popular venue to find sexual partners among high-risk individuals for HIV infection who are unlikely to seek medical attention due to the lack of information on testing or feeling of shame, or stigmatization. Anonymous and voluntary counseling services within partner-finding websites greatly lowered barrier to clinic visits [56]. Socioeconomically disadvantaged and stigmatized individuals now have a greater opportunity to seek and access relevant health information and resources.

2.3 Online Surveillance

Although the Internet is becoming a primary media for health information seeking and communication among youth [55, 57], it is a highly unregulated environment filled with information lacking credibility and legitimacy and became an important channel for marketing of unhealthy products (and thus behaviors) created by industries. For instance, discussion of alcohol consumption in youth SNS communities is manipulated towards pro-drinking by alcohol industries [58]. Twitter is an important tool for marketing e-cigarettes, with overwhelmingly positive messages generated for commercial intent [40, 59, 60]. Industries are far ahead of realizing the value of social media in pursuing consumer behaviors, with established tactics such as creating online "viral" messages [62].

Governments cannot freely regulate the contents of the Internet unless information pose a clear threat to the health of public. However, continuous monitoring of online health information and its potential impact on health-related behavior is necessary. Given the growing importance of the Internet as a source of health information, facilitating access to credible information will be beneficial to the public. This is particularly relevant to individuals suffering chronic health conditions who may desperately seek expert advice [63, 64]. Finally, social media is an important venue to identify a new generation of public health issues including online bullying, sexual solicitation, and depression from SNS use [40].

3 Ethical Challenges in the Use of Big Data and the Web 2.0 Technologies

Lack of appropriate regulation on collection and analysis of personal data by industry and government surveillance resulted in public concerns about the loss of privacy and autonomy and profiling of citizens [21, 65]. Tracking online customer activities (often secretly to users) became industry-wide practice. Personally, identifiable data is routinely collected, centralized, and permanently stored by search engines and social networking sites (SNS) and undergoes mass disclosure (i.e., sold to their parties) without users' permission and even awareness [66]. Such data is in turn used to predict personally sensitive attributes including sexual orientation, political view, parental separation [21, 67] and to generate personalized advertisement aimed at driving consumer preference and decision [68]. In addition, widespread sharing of personal information on the Internet poses a unique challenge in defining online privacy [69, 70]. Users self-disclosing personal information in SNS or blogs typically expect their messages to be exposed to the online world. However, it does not imply that the data is subject to amassing and indiscriminate use, as such activities can lead to reidentification and potential harm to the users [70], which certainly conflict with the users' expectation [69]. Individuals who are affected by stigmatizing illness particularly express concerns with the unintended use of their data by third parties [71]. Despite the public nature of social media, privacy does exist as a right to prevent data usage that leads to stigmatization, restriction of liberty, and violation of privacy.

Some users publish their health and non-health information openly due to the sheer lack of privacy concerns and awareness. Such users are unlikely to be familiar with the contents of the privacy policies and statements in social media, which may state the usage of personal information by third parties. Even if users attempt to read privacy statements, inconsistency and complexity of privacy settings and policies in ever-growing social media applications make controlling of personal information far from trivial [72–74]. Yet, the legitimacy of these policies without users' explicit understanding in terms of risks and benefits is highly questionable. Therefore, sharing of sensitive information in the online environment does not necessarily equate to consent for data usage. Furthermore, it is not clear whether the data usage policies in these websites encompass public health surveillance. Although public health agencies are exempt from obtaining consent for secondary use of patient health records, such action is justifiable only in the presence of clear and immediate public health risk [11].

3.1 Profiling and Predictive Analytics

Predictive analysis can be performed at both individual and community levels for predicting of future health-related attributes (e.g., diseases, prognosis, behaviors, and resource utilization), or inferring unobserved health-related attributes status as in disease diagnosis. Rapid increase and linking of personal, social and environmental information from a large number of individuals in the Internet provide a sufficient set of predictive features for an accurate inference of sensitive personal attributes [75] such as body mass index, depression, emotion, sexual orientation, personality, and various behaviors [76–78].

Because predictive features are not directly collected from individuals but often accumulated in organizations running such algorithms, the targeted individuals have little control over the use of their information against the prediction of their personal or community attributes. These predicted personal features can be highly sensitive and potentially used in ways to damage their liberty and reputation [75]. The indiscriminate use of predictive algorithms can open a potential avenue to a public health analog of "predictive policing", where health agencies could target, contact, and impose restrictive interventions on individuals with heightened risk of developing highly pathogenic communicable disease or behavior (e.g., violence and illicit drug use) of public health significance.

Similar to medical screening, these algorithms can facilitate early identification and notification of potentially serious health condition(s) to facilitate effective prevention measures. However, "black box" algorithm-based diagnosis and risk prediction from online data sources are qualitatively distinct from screening. Unlike screening test which are typically performed with informed participation, predictive algorithms can secretly profile millions of social media users without awareness of those who are targeted. Accidental or intentional disclosure of their predicted disease status can affect socioeconomic status including employment and insurance, whereas prediction of highly personal characteristic such as sexual orientation can be intrinsically offending. Excessive use of predictive algorithms to generate a large repository of sensitive characteristics can be highly concerning. It is therefore challenging for individuals to escape from the privacy assault from prediction and resist presumptive activities and automatic profiling by the government [79, 80] especially in the face of automatic data collection by ubiquitous sensor devices (e.g., including mobile smart phones), with their often opt-out nature of data submission.

Application of predictive algorithm at a community or group level, in general, prevents privacy harm at individual level due to aggregation; however, profiling and ranking communities by future disease burden may lead to public discomfort and label high-risk communities (e.g., high prevalence of smoking, obesity, or alcohol consumption) as a potential burden for a society. Community health profiling based on traditional data sources, such as population health survey, has been a routine task of health department. However, prediction of future community health by a data-driven approach undermines the fundamental value of "right to know" for citizens, potentially causing distrust to health authorities. At worst, the fear of being labeled by such algorithms will lead privacy-sensitive individuals to avoid the use of social media, whereas those lacking privacy and technology literacy will give up all their personal attributes to the intrusive activity of predictive algorithms.

3.2   New Age of Digital Divide

Although diminishing steadily, digital divide impedes fair distribution of technological benefits throughout the society. Individuals lacking connectivity to the Internet may be protected from data gathering activities of government and industries; however, their needs and voices may be underrepresented in the online society, resulting in interventions not reflecting their socioeconomic and cultural needs and interests.

An emerging and equally important form of technological disparity is a gap in usage purpose and capability to make effective use of online content for informed health-related decision-making [45, 81, 82]. Even with the Internet access, those at the lower level of educational attainment are less likely to use the online contents for the enrichment of their socioeconomic resources (e.g., beneficial information to promote career, education, and social position) and health information seeking [83, 84]. One of the main factors driving this usage gap, or secondary-level digital divide, is a lack of technology literacy among individuals with low socioeconomic status [64, 85].

However, the usage gap appears to exist even if conditioned on technological literacy, suggesting the presence of motivational factor(s) [83]. Although such differential usage may have existed in traditional media including newspapers and televisions, the amount and diversity of information on the Internet are far greater, thereby resulting in a potentially larger inequality in terms of benefit from the Internet across social classes [83]. If the usage pattern of the Internet has a stronger reflection of existing socioeconomic status than the usage pattern of traditional media, simple reliance on technology-based interventions may lead to the exacerbation of socioeconomic disparity in health-related knowledge and behaviors and other gains from Internet-based interventions.

At the international level, borderless nature of digital data could inadvertently introduce inequity across nations as well when used in global health surveillance. For example, data generated in low and middle-income countries is often analyzed in research labs and public health organizations in developed nations with little or limited return to the population health in the countries of origin, who may be eventually discouraged to share information in the event of an international health crisis [86].

4   Discussions

Used effectively, researchers and public health agencies can harness the power of Big Data and Web 2.0 technologies to meet the expanding responsibility of public health and improve the community and individual health. If, however, their ethical challenges remain unaddressed, public distrust and opposition can prevent the utilization of potentially useful technologies and dataset, thereby limiting the capacity of public health agencies in the future. One of the challenges lies in the speed of technological advancement and their potential applications that could far exceed the pace legislation can catch up. Nevertheless, there is an urgent need to discuss the development of tactics to facilitate their implementation into public health practice.

In this section, we explore key aspects of Big Data and Web 2.0 applications/services needed for (*i*) minimization of privacy harm; (*ii*) fair distribution of benefit; and (*iii*) transparency and user engagement.

4.1 Privacy and Confidentiality

Given the growing concerns over the intense data gathering activities by government and industries [87], public acceptance towards the application of social media and mobile technologies hinges to adequate assurance of privacy and confidentiality. Currently, existing local public health laws about the collection, storage, and sharing of electronic health data are inconsistent and incomplete, and typically require major review and reform to reflect the growing use of electronic personal information [18]. In addition, the challenge of defining privacy in online personal information makes the protection of privacy even more complex [88]. Attempts to seek privacy solution are scarce [71, 88], yet urgently needed.

Policy

Guidelines for security, privacy, and confidentiality concerning the use of personally identifiable information under public health purpose have been subject to discussion. Although these discussions do not specifically address the application of online personal information but more often limited to patient data generated and maintained by healthcare organizations, they are broadly applicable to the secondary use of personally identifiable information in the online environment. Specifically, the amount of personal information collected should be the minimum necessary to meet the well-defined goal of surveillance and the disease control program [89]. The openness of the Internet and rapidly lowering cost of data storage can create a temptation for large-scale collection, process, and centralization of personal information. Such practice, if not guided by clearly defined usage purpose, will introduce a predictable risk of reidentification [9].

Public release of findings from surveillance programs (i.e., reports) requires appropriate de-identification measures such as data aggregation to prevent reidentification and should be subject to automated or manual review prior to dissemination [90]. If findings are related to stigmatizing diseases, a prior consultation with affected communities is needed to prevent stigmatization and discrimination. Unfortunately, no de-identification method can assure complete anonymity as the linkage to a large number of external and publicly available data can lead to reidentification of individual [91, 92]. Therefore, the definition of anonymity needs to be treated as continuous scale [21], with the privacy risk of individuals carefully balanced against the health of population achieved by public health programs.

Moreover, limitation of the scale and scope of data collections and disclosure needs to be clearly specified even during public health crisis such as the emergence of highly pathogenic communicable diseases. The exemption from obtaining ethics review and patients' consent to access personal health information opens up unlimited authority for data access and potentially results in an excess level of intrusive activities [93]. However, the totalitarian measures of disease control do not guarantee success, while public disapproval and outcry are certain, which potentially pushes back the utilization of the modern data science technology in public health.

Privacy by Design and Education

Confidentiality policies need to be accompanied by organizational practice, which can be achieved by training of employee who has access to data and the implementation of preventive technologies. Rigorous authentication and authorization protocols play a primary role in restricting inappropriate data release. These include multiple modes of authentication, the minimum necessary number of personnel with data access, physical restriction to workstations and servers, and periodic review of access privileges. Encryption of data transfer and communications is another necessary system-wide security measure, particularly when remote access to data sources is required. In addition, any personal information in the data center should be accessed by authorized individuals only on the need-to-know basis.

Most breaches of personal health information are unintentional and occur internally within health organizations as opposed to the external cause with the malicious purpose [18]. Effective prevention of data breach can be achieved by enhancing vigilance in handling personal information through confidentiality agreements with data analysists. They need to be properly informed the consequences of inappropriate disclosure including disciplinary actions. Furthermore, routine auditing of data usage will allow the detection of breach and malpractice as well as provide an enforcement and awareness for privacy-conscious activities.

Information Control

Whether one's data is intended to be viewed by public or peers, assurance of information privacy requires that consumers have control over their personal attributes in terms of what information to share with whom for what purpose, in addition to receiving adequate information about privacy policy in the Web 2.0 applications/services. Ideally, these controls encompass the amount and type of information for location-based analysis, spatiotemporal context, and the recipients and users of such data as well as access to the result of analysis [88].

Unfortunately, low availability, readability (e.g., excessive text), and interpretability (e.g., legal terms) of policy statements even among commonly used applications deter the consumers and consequently leave them blind with privacy risks [66, 73]. In addition, there are common misconceptions about the policy in social networks, such as the lack of complete understanding in the "permanency" of recorded data and the false sense of security from reidentification among Twitter users [71]. As well, many users wrongly interpret the presence of a privacy policy as the assurance for the protection of their personal data, even though the policy statements do not always describe privacy protection [94]. Therefore, users often fail to set the appropriate level of disclosure, resulting in unintended disclosure of their own and others' sensitive information [95, 96]. A clear privacy policy in terms of confidentiality rules, usage, and sharing of personal information by service providers and third parties is needed, and such information should be provided in the sixth-grade reading level [73]. In addition, standardization of terminology and formats of privacy statements should be implemented across providers/developers of health applications [97].

4.2 Population Reach and Engagement

Improvement in citizen engagement and population reach is crucial for effective dissemination of public health interventions and maintaining representative population in public health surveillances. Specifically, strong public engagement and collaboration can ensure accurate data quality and prevent loss to follow up in longitudinal data collection. On the other hand, wider population outreach facilitates the inclusion of underserved and hard-to-reach individuals.

Although the primary level of digital divide (i.e., lack of access to the Internet) may continue to decline due to the widespread use of mobile devices, the gap remains important for certain population subgroups, such as those who live in the rural area [45, 51]. Providing communication infrastructure and affordability of Internet access to these communities requires public/private collaboration and government subsidization [85]. In addition, lack of access among socioeconomically disadvantaged population persists in many developing nations [85], where providing shared connection at community access center may provide an only viable solution [98].

Narrowing the secondary level of digital divide (i.e., usage pattern of the Internet among those who have access) will at minimum require improvement of technology and health literacy, which may encourage active participation (e.g., sharing information, peer to peer communication, and seeking credible health-related information) [64, 85]. At the same time, the complexity and amount of information should be minimum necessary to meet the need for users with a minimum level of health literacy [45]. Because usage gap may also depend on factors beyond literacy (e.g., sociocultural preference) [83], further research is needed to explore such barriers and to identify approaches aimed at motivating Internet usage for the empowerment of health-related behaviors and information seeking.

Evaluation of behavioral change through the Web 2.0 applications/services has been relying on a small-scale randomized trial [34, 99]. However, study population from small trials do not adequately represent the heterogeneous needs of general population, particularly when measuring the performance of interventions among underserved and underprivileged population segments who may be less likely to participate into these studies due to the lack of access to the Internet or motivation for participation. Large-scale trials with the minimization of attrition or natural experiment will provide the best evidence needed to identify equitable quality and effectiveness of Internet-delivered interventions.

To date, the majority of research studies investigating the applications of social media have not been completely successful to exploit the "social" component; rather, researchers tended to treat SNS as a mere broadcasting tool that does not incorporate tailoring of messages meeting the diverse socioeconomic and cultural context of users [48, 99, 100]. Simply focusing on unidirectional communications ignoring the interactivity, tailoring, and peer engagement is likely to add little value over traditional communication channels. Efforts should be allocated towards leveraging the user-centric features of participatory applications to meet heterogeneous needs of population subgroups, and the tailored messaging should encourage informed decision-making for people with varying language, cultural background, disability, health and technological literacy and numeracy [101–103]. With the media-rich feature of the Internet, messages can be conveyed by the combination of images and video for the latter users for enhanced uptake [45].

Properly crafted health message and engaging environment will be an effective instrument to empower individuals, especially those with stigmatizing illness, who are more likely to use the Internet to seek health information and peer support [49, 104]. However, given the fact that health promotion messages can be amplified and escalate to the public ridicule of individuals suffering from potentially stigmatizing conditions, contents should be delivered in such a way to minimize stereotyping, while facilitating the active participation and empowerment of these individuals [49].

4.3 Transparency

Public health is a societal effort requiring active citizen engagement, which demands transparency of public health practices and decision-making process. Transparency implies timely dissemination of information related to the process of data collection and analysis, purpose, risks (e.g., privacy issues), and benefits of surveillance [105]. For public health interventions, all levels of relevant decision process (i.e., planning, implementation, operation, evaluation, and public reporting) should be available to the public. Providing such information to disadvantaged individuals and communities who are often least likely to benefit from public health actions [71, 105] is particularly an important task towards increasing the transparency.

Informing community is especially important when using publicly available online data since (*i*) public perception of Big Data analytics may have been transformed from "creepy practice" to actual privacy threatening after the previous revelation of government surveillance and industry practice conducted largely unknown to public [65, 106]; (*ii*) inappropriate use of such data will result in more serious damage to privacy and autonomy of individuals due to a large population coverage of digital data; and (*iii*) surveillance programs and predictive algorithms processing unstructured online data often require complex analysis, which is beyond understanding of lay community members. The feeling of being monitored and profiled by a "black box algorithm" can cause serious distress among people.

One of the major benefits of public disclosure is to prevent illegitimate and unjustified use, manipulation, and distribution of personal information by health departments while facilitating the minimum necessary data collection and analysis for specific and intended purpose only [21]. Finally, in anticipation of a public health crisis (e.g., bioterrorism and emerging infectious agent of pandemic potential) and the resulting use of authoritative power for effective emergency response, it is critical to specify appropriate safeguards for individual rights and due process [107]. Despite unavoidable risk on privacy, patients and the general public would allow the secondary use of their data for surveillance; however, such trust is unlikely to be cultivated unless the transparency showing the rationale of the monitoring program is provided [61].

5   Conclusions

Successful application of Big Data will provide enhanced capabilities for disease surveillance and dissemination of public health interventions. Public health surveillance can also benefit from the data stream generated by a large number of sentinel citizen, and ubiquitous nature of Web 2.0 applications/services which enable increased population outreach. The interactive and collaborative characteristics of the Web 2.0 applications/services are likely to enhance citizen engagement with health interventions and encourage proactive contribution of user information to public health surveillance. In addition, the anonymity of the Internet provides a protection from stigmatization and stereotyping when communicating with public health agencies or among peers.

However, the utilization of these technologies will be justifiable only if accompanied with a clear ethical framework and guideline. Applications of Big Data are still in their infancy, and the impact on public health practice is yet to be revealed. However, it is crucial to explore the potential benefits and harms at the earliest opportunity to avoid repeating the lessons learned from industries and to maximize its utility for the public good.

References

1. Kass, N.E.: An Ethics framework for public health. Am. J. Public Health **91**, 1776–1782 (2001)
2. Perdue, W.C., Stone, L.A., Gostin, L.O.: The built environment and its relationship to the public's health: the legal framework. Am. J. Public Health **93**(9), 1390–1394 (2003)
3. Prevention, C.D.C.: Achievements in public health, 1900–1999: control of infectious diseases. JAMA **283**(3), 621–629 (1999)
4. World Health Organization.: Global status report on noncommunicable diseases 2014. (2014)
5. Dayan, G.H., Quinlisk, M.P., Parker, A.A., Barskey, A.E., Harris, M.L., Schwartz, J.M.H., Hunt, K., Finley, C.G., Leschinsky, D.P., O'Keefe, A.L., Clayton, J., Kightlinger, L.K., Dietle, E.G., Berg, J., Kenyon, C., Goldstein, S.T., Stokley, S.K., Redd, S.B., Rota, P.A., Rota, J., Bi, D., Roush, S.W., Bridges, C.B., Santibanez, T.A., Parashar, U., Bellini, W.J., Seward, J.F.: Recent resurgence of mumps in the United States. N. Engl. J. Med. **358**(15), 1580–1589 (2008)
6. Porteous, G.H., Hanson, N.A., Sueda, L.A., Hoaglan, C.D., Dahl, A.B., Ohlson, B.B., Schmid, B.E., Wang, C.C., Fagley, R.E.: Resurgence of vaccine-preventable diseases in the United States: anesthetic and critical care implications. Anesth. Analg. **122**(5), 1450–1473 (2016)
7. WHO Ebola Response Team, Agua-Agum, J., Allegranzi, B., Ariyarajah, A., Aylward, R., Blake IM, Barboza P, Bausch D, Brennan, R.J., Clement, P, Coffey, P., Cori, A., Donnelly, C.A., Dorigatti, I., Drury, P., Durski, K., Dye, C., Eckmanns, T., Ferguson, N.M., Fraser, C., Garcia, E., Garske, T., Gasasira, A., Gurry, C., Hamblion, E., Hinsley, W., Holden, R., Holmes, D., Hugonnet, S., Jaramillo, G.G., Jombart, T., Kelley, E., Santhana, R., Mahmoud, N., Mills, H.L., Mohamed, Y., Musa, E., Naidoo, D., Nedjati-Gilani, G., Newton, E., Norton, I., Nouvellet, P., Perkins, D., Perkins, M., Riley, S., Schumacher, D., Shah, A., Tang, M., Varsaneux, O., Van Kerkhove, M.D.: After Ebola in West Africa–unpredictable risks, preventable epidemics. New England J. Med. **375**(6), 587–596 (2016)
8. Gostin, L.O.: Public health law and ethics. A reader. 2 ed. University of California Press, California (2010)
9. Lee, L.M., Heilig, C.M., White, A.: Ethical justification for conducting public health surveillance without patient consent. Am. J. Public Health **102**(1), 38–44 (2012)
10. Fairchild, A.L., Bayer, R., Colgrove, J.: Privacy, democracy and the politics of disease surveillance. Public Health Ethics. **1**(1), 30–38 (2008)
11. Fairchild, A.L., Bayer, R.: Public health. Ethics and the conduct of public health surveillance. Science **303**(5658), 631–632 (2004)
12. Carter, S.M., Cribb, A., Allegrante, J.P.: How to think about health promotion ethics. Public Health Rev. **34**(9), 1–24 (2012)
13. Public Health Law and Ethics: A reader. 2 ed. University of California Press, California (2010)
14. Jones, M.M., Bayer, R.: Paternalism & its discontents: motorcycle helmet laws, libertarian values, and public health. Am. J. Public Health **97**(2), 208–217 (2007)
15. Lee, L.M., Gostin, L.O.: Ethical collection, storage, and use of public health data: a proposal for a national privacy protection. JAMA **302**(1), 82–84 (2009)
16. Fairchild, A.L., Alkon, A.: Back to the future? Diabetes, HIV, and the boundaries of public health. J. Health Polit. Policy Law **32**(4), 561–593 (2007)
17. O'Brien, D.G., Yasnoff, W.A.: Privacy, confidentiality, and security in information systems of state health agencies. Am. J. Prev. Med. **16**(4), 351–358 (1999)
18. Myers, J., Frieden, T.R., Bherwani, K.M., Henning, K.J.: Ethics in public health research: privacy and public health at risk: public health confidentiality in the digital age. Am. J. Public Health **98**(5), 793–801 (2008)

19. Provost, F., Fawcett, T.: Data science and its relationship to big data and data-driven decision making. Big Data. **1**(1), 51–59 (2013)
20. Erl, T., Khattak, W., Buhler, P.: Big Data Fundamentals: Concepts, Drivers and Techniques. Prentice Hall Press, Englewood 240 p (2016)
21. Omer Tene JP. Big data for all: Privacy and user control in the age of analytics. Northwest. J. Technol. Intellect. Property. **11**(5), 239–273 (2013)
22. Boyd, D., Crawford, K.: Critical questions for big data. Inf. Commun. Soc. **15**(5), 662–79 (2012)
23. Davis, K.: Ethics of big data: balancing risk and innovation. O'Reilly Media (2012)
24. Wilder-James, E.: What is big data? O'Reilly Media, Inc. 2012. Retrieved on July 10, 2017. http://strata.oreilly.com/2012/01/what-is-big-data.html
25. O'Reilly, T.: What is Web 2.0: Design patterns and business models for the next generation of software. Commun. Strat. **1**(7/July/2017), 17–37 (2005)
26. Eysenbach, G.: Infodemiology and infoveillance tracking online health information and cyberbehavior for public health. Am. J. Prev. Med. **40**(5 Suppl 2), S154–S158 (2011)
27. Kass-Hout, T.A., Alhinnawi, H.: Social media in public health. Br. Med. Bull. **108**(1), 5–24 (2013)
28. Pentland, A., Lazer, D., Brewer, D., Heibeck, T.: Using reality mining to improve public health and medicine. Stud. Health Technol. Inform. **149**, 93–102 (2009)
29. Wyber, R., Vaillancourt, S., Perry, W., Mannava, P., Folaranmi, T., Celi, L.A.: Big data in global health: improving health in low- and middle-income countries. Bull. World Health Organ. **93**(3), 203–208 (2015)
30. Oldenburg, B., Taylor, C.B., O'Neil, A., Cocker, F., Cameron, L.D.: Using new technologies to improve the prevention and management of chronic conditions in populations. Annu. Rev. Public Health **36**, 483–505 (2015)
31. Brinkel, J., Krämer, A., Krumkamp, R., May, J., Fobil, J.: Mobile phone-based mhealth approaches for public health surveillance in Sub-Saharan Africa: a systematic review. Int. J. Environ. Res. Public Health. **11**(11), 11559–11582 (2014)
32. Conway, M.: Ethical issues in using Twitter for public health surveillance and research: developing a taxonomy of ethical concepts from the research literature. J. Med. Internet Res. **16**, e290 (2014)
33. Pew Research Center. Few See Adequate Limits on NSA Surveillance Program 2013 [updated 2013-07-26]
34. Oldenburg, B., Taylor, C.B., O'Neil, A., Cocker, F., Cameron, L.D.: Using new technologies to improve the prevention and management of chronic conditions in populations. Annu. Rev. Public Health **36**(1), 483–505 (2015)
35. Harris, J.K., Moreland-Russell, S., Choucair, B., Mansour, R., Staub, M., Simmons, K.: Tweeting for and against public health policy: response to the Chicago Department of Public Health's electronic cigarette Twitter Campaign. J. Med. Internet Res. **16**, e238 (2014)
36. Baskerville, N.B., Struik, L.L., Hammond, D., Guindon, G.E., Norman, C.D., Whittaker, R., Burns, C.M., Grindrod, K.A., Brown, K.S.: Effect of a mobile phone intervention on quitting smoking in a young adult population of smokers: randomized controlled trial study protocol. JMIR Res. Protoc. **4**(1), e10 (2015)
37. Brownstein, J.S., Freifeld, C.C., Madoff, L.C.: Digital disease detection—harnessing the web for public health surveillance. N. Engl. J. Med. **360**(21), 2153–2157 (2009)
38. Hay, S.I., George, D.B., Moyes, C.L., Brownstein, J.S.: Big data opportunities for global infectious disease surveillance. PLoS Med. **10**(4), e1001413 (2013)
39. Wong, C.A., Merchant, R.M., Moreno, M.A.: Using social media to engage adolescents and young adults with their health. Healthcare. **2**(4), 220–224 (2014)
40. Capurro, D., Cole, K., Echavarría, M.I., Joe, J., Neogi, T., Turner, A.M.: The use of social networking sites for public health practice and research: a systematic review. J. Med. Internet Res. **16**(3), e79 (2014)

41. Yang, C., Yang, J., Luo, X., Gong, P.: Use of mobile phones in an emergency reporting system for infectious disease surveillance after the Sichuan earthquake in China. Bull. World Health Organ. **87**, 619–623 (2008)
42. Hudnut-Beumler, J., Po'e, E., Barkin, S.: The use of social media for health promotion in hispanic populations: a scoping systematic review. JMIR Public Health Surveill. **2**(2), e32 (2016)
43. Gibbons, M.C., Fleisher, L., Slamon, R.E., Bass, S., Kandadai, V., Beck, J.R.: Exploring the potential of Web 2.0 to address health disparities. J. Health Commun. **16**(Suppl 1), 77–89 (2011)
44. Eysenbach, G.: Medicine 2.0: social networking, collaboration, participation, apomediation, and openness. J. Med. Internet Res. **10**(3), e22 (2008)
45. Chou, W.Y., Prestin, A., Lyons, C., Wen, K.Y.: Web 2.0 for health promotion: reviewing the current evidence. Am. J. Public Health **103**(1), e9–e18 (2013)
46. Crawford, R.: You are dangerous to your health: the ideology and politics of victim blaming. Int. J. Health Serv. Plan. Adm. Eval. **7**(4), 663–680 (1977)
47. Couch, D., Thomas, S.L., Lewis, S., Blood, R.W., Komesaroff, P.: Obese adults' perceptions of news reporting on obesity. the panopticon and synopticon at work. Sage Open **5**(4), 2158244015612522 (2015)
48. Heldman, A.B., Schindelar, J., Weaver III, J.B.: Social media engagement and public health communication: implications for public health organizations being truly "Social". Public Health Rev. **35**(1), 1–18 (2013)
49. Lewis, S., Thomas, S.L., Blood, R.W., Castle, D., Hyde, J., Komesaroff, P.A.: 'I'm searching for solutions': why are obese individuals turning to the Internet for help and support with 'being fat'? Health Expect. Int. J. Public Participation Health Care Health Policy. **14**(4), 339–350 (2011)
50. Gallagher, S., Doherty, D.T.: Searching for health information online: characteristics of online health seekers. J. Evid. Based Med. **2**(2), 99–106 (2009)
51. Pew Research Center. Americans' Internet Access: 2000–2015 Washington, D.C. 2015. Retrieved on July 10, 2017. http://www.pewinternet.org/2015/06/26/americans-internet-access-2000-2015/
52. Pew Research Center. U.S. Smartphone use in 2015 Washington, D.C. 2015. Retrieved on July 10, 2017. http://www.pewinternet.org/2015/04/01/us-smartphone-use-in-2015/
53. Pew Research Center. Smartphone ownership and internet usage continues to climb in emerging economies Washington, D.C. 2016. Retrieved on July 10, 2017. http://www.pewglobal.org/2016/02/22/smartphone-ownership-and-internet-usage-continues-to-climb-in-emerging-economies/
54. Kontos, E.Z., Emmons, K.M., Puleo, E., Viswanath, K.: Communication inequalities and public health implications of adult social networking site use in the United States. J. Health Commun. **15**(Suppl 3), 216–235 (2010)
55. Laranjo, L., Arguel, A., Neves, A.L., Gallagher, A.M., Kaplan, R., Mortimer, N., et al.: The influence of social networking sites on health behavior change: a systematic review and meta-analysis. J. Am. Med. Inform. Assoc. JAMIA. **22**(1), 243–256 (2015)
56. Feldacker, C., Torrone, E., Triplette, M., Smith, J.C., Leone, P.A.: Reaching and retaining high-risk HIV/AIDS clients through the internet. Health Promot. Pract. **12**(4), 522–528 (2011)
57. Watson, R., Wyness, L.: 'Don't tell me what to eat!'—ways to engage the population in positive behaviour change. Nutr. Bulletin. **38**(1), 23–29 (2013)
58. Griffiths, R., Casswell, S.: Intoxigenic digital spaces? Youth, social networking sites and alcohol marketing. Drug Alcohol Rev. **29**(5), 525–530 (2010)
59. Huang, J., Kornfield, R., Szczypka, G., Emery, S.L.: A cross-sectional examination of marketing of electronic cigarettes on Twitter. Tob. Control **23**, iii26–iii30 (2014)
60. Moorhead, S.A., Hazlett, D.E., Harrison, L., Carroll, J.K., Irwin, A., Hoving, C.: A new dimension of health care: systematic review of the uses, benefits, and limitations of social media for health communication. J. Med. Internet Res. **15**(4), e85 (2013)

61. Kohane, I.S., Altman, R.B.: Health-information altruists—a potentially critical resource. N. Engl. J. Med. **353**, 2074–2077 (2005)
62. Freeman, B., Chapman, S.: Gone viral? Heard the buzz? A guide for public health practitioners and researchers on how Web 2.0 can subvert advertising restrictions and spread health information. J. Epidemiol. Community Health **62**, 778–782 (2008)
63. Ostry, A., Young, M.L., Hughes, M.: The quality of nutritional information available on popular websites: a content analysis. Health Educ. Res. **23**(4), 648–655 (2008)
64. McCloud, R.F., Okechukwu, C.A., Sorensen, G., Viswanath, K.: Beyond access: barriers to internet health information seeking among the urban poor. J. Am. Med. Inform. Assoc. **23** (6), 1053–1059 (2016)
65. Pew Research Center.: Public perceptions of privacy and security in the Post-Snowden Era Washington, D.C. 2014. Retrieved on July 10, 2017. http://www.pewinternet.org/2014/11/12/public-privacy-perceptions/
66. Li, J.: Privacy policies for health social networking sites. J. Am. Med. Inform. Assoc. **20**, 704–707 (2013)
67. The Center for Media Justice. Consumers, big data, and online tracking in the retail industry: a case study of Walmart. Center for Media Justice, ColorOfChange, Sum of Us 2013. Retrieved July 10, 2017. centerformediajustice.org/wp-content/uploads/2014/06/walmart_privacy_pdf
68. Jerome, J.: Buying and selling privacy: big data's different burdens and benefits. SSRN Scholarly Paper. Social Science Research Network, Rochester, NY, 2013/06/30/. Report No.: ID 2294996
69. McKee, R.: Ethical issues in using social media for health and health care research. Health Policy **110**(2–3), 298–301 (2013)
70. Small, H., Kasianovitz, K., Blanford, R., Celaya, I.: What your tweets tell us about you: identity, ownership and privacy of twitter data. Int. J. Digit. Curation **7**(1), 174–197 (2012)
71. Mikal, J., Hurst, S., Conway, M.: Ethical issues in using Twitter for population-level depression monitoring: a qualitative study. BMC Med. Ethics. **17**, 22 (2016)
72. Society I. Global Internet Report 2015.: Mobile evolution and development of the internet. 2015. Retrieved on July 10, 2017. http://www.internetsociety.org/globalinternetreport/2015/assets/download/IS_web.pdf
73. Sunyaev, A., Dehling, T., Taylor, P.L., Mandl, K.D.: Availability and quality of mobile health app privacy policies. J. Am. Med. Inform. Assoc. **22**(e1), e28–e33 (2015)
74. McDonald, A.A., Cranor, L.F.: The cost of reading privacy policies. J. Law Policy Inf. Soc. **4**(3), 540–565 (2012)
75. Crawford, K., Schultz, J.: Big data and due process: toward a framework to redress predictive privacy harms. SSRN Scholarly Paper. Rochester, NY: Social Science Research Network 2013/10/01/. Report No.: ID 2325784
76. Wen, L., Guodong, G.A.: computational approach to body mass index prediction from face images. Image Vis. Comput. **31**(5), 392–400 (2013)
77. Kosinski, M., Stillwell, D., Graepel, T.: Private traits and attributes are predictable from digital records of human behavior. Proc. Natl. Acad. Sci. U S A. **110**(15), 5802–5805 (2013)
78. Duhigg, C.: How Companies learn your secrets: the New York Times; 2012. Retrieved on July 10, 2017. http://www.nytimes.com/2012/02/19/magazine/shopping-habits.html
79. Ian Kerr, J.E.: Prediction preemption, presumption: how big data threatens big picture privacy. Stanford Law Rev. Online **66**, 65–71 (2013)
80. The Government of Canada.: Office of the Privacy Commissioner of Canada. The Age of Predictive Analytics: From Patterns to Predictions Ottawa, On: Government of Canada; 2013 [updated 2013-09-17; cited 2016 26-Sep_2016]. Retrieved on July 10, 2017. https://www.priv.gc.ca/en/opc-actions-and-decisions/research/explore-privacy-research/2012/pa_201208/#toc_e5d
81. Büchi, M., Just, N., Latzer, M.: Modeling the second-level digital divide: a five-country study of social differences in Internet use. New Media Soc. **18**(11), 2703–2722 (2015)

82. Pew Research Center.: Digital readiness gaps Washington, D.C. 2015. Retrieved on July 10, 2017. http://www.pewinternet.org/2016/09/20/digital-readiness-gaps/
83. van Deursen, A.J., van Dijk, J.A.: The digital divide shifts to differences in usage. New Media & Society. **16**(3), 507–526 (2014)
84. Pollard, C.M., Pulker, C.E., Meng, X., Kerr, D.A., Scott, J.A.: Who uses the internet as a source of nutrition and dietary information? An Australian population perspective. J. Med. Internet Res. **17**(8), e209 (2015)
85. Rowena, C.: Addressing the digital divide. Online Inf. Rev. **25**(5), 311–320 (2001)
86. Brack, M., Edelstein, M., Herten-Crabb, A., Harper, D.R.: Openness, transparency and equity in public health surveillance data sharing. Online J. Public Health Inf. **8**(1) (2016)
87. Pew Research Center.: Americans' attitudes about privacy, security and surveillance 2015 [updated 2016-02-19]. Retrieved on July 10, 2017. http://www.pewinternet.org/2015/05/20/americans-attitudes-about-privacy-security-and-surveillance/
88. Christin, D., Reinhardt, A., Kanhere, S.S., Hollick, M.: A survey on privacy in mobile participatory sensing applications. J. Syst. Softw. **84**(11), 1928–1946 (2011)
89. Glynn, M.K., Backer, L.C.: Collecting public health surveillance data: creating a surveillance system. In: Lee L.M., Teutsch, S.M., Thacker, S.B., St. Louis, M.E. (eds.) Principles & Practice of Public Health Surveillance, 3rd ed. England (2010)
90. Yasnoff, W.A.: Privacy, confidentiality, and security of public health information. In: O'Carroll, P.W., Ripp, L.H., Yasnoff, W.A., Ward, E., Martin, E.L. (eds.) Public Health Informatics and Information Systems. Springer, New York (2003)
91. Ohm, P.: Broken promises of privacy: Responding to the surprising failure of anonymization. UCLA Law Rev. **57**, 1701 (2009)
92. de Montjoye, Y.A., Hidalgo, C.A., Verleysen, M., Blondel, V.D.: Unique in the crowd: The privacy bounds of human mobility. Sci. Rep. **3**, 1376 (2013)
93. Fairchild, A.L., Bayyer, R., Colgrove, J.: Panoptic visions and stubborn realities in a New Era of privacy. In: Fairchild, A.L, Bayyer, R., Colgrove, J. (eds.) Searching Eyes New York: University of California Press, Milbank Memorial Fund (2007)
94. Turow, D.K.M., Hoofnagle, C.J.: Research Report: Consumers Fundamentally Misunderstand the Online Advertising Marketplace. School of Law, University of California, Berkeley, CA (2007)
95. Madejski, M., Johnson, M., Bellovin, S.M. (eds.): A study of privacy settings errors in an online social network. 2012 IEEE International Conference on Pervasive Computing and Communications Workshops; 19–23 March 2012
96. MacDonald, J., Sohn, S., Ellis, P.: Privacy, professionalism and Facebook: a dilemma for young doctors. Med. Educ. **44**(8), 805–813 (2010)
97. FTC Staff Report.: Mobile privacy disclosures: building trust through transparency. February 2013. Retrieved on July 10, 2017. https://law.ku.edu/sites/law.ku.edu/files/docs/media_law/Mobile_Privacy_Disclosures.pdf
98. Hilbert, M.: When is cheap, cheap enough to bridge the digital divide? Modeling income related structural challenges of technology diffusion in Latin America. World Dev. **38**(5), 756–770 (2010)
99. Bennett, G.G., Glasgow, R.E.: The delivery of public health interventions via the Internet: actualizing their potential. Annu. Rev. Public Health **30**, 273–292 (2009)
100. Clar, C., Dyakova, M., Curtis, K., Dawson, C., Donnelly, P., Knifton, L., Clarke, A.: Just telling and selling: current limitations in the use of digital media in public health: a scoping review. Public Health. **128**, 1066–1075 (2014)
101. Lazarus, W., Mora, F.: Online Content for Low-Income and Underserved Americans: The Digital Divide's New Frontier. The Children's Partnership, Santa Monica, CA (2000)
102. López, L., Grant, R.W.: Closing the gap: Eliminating Health care disparities among latinos with diabetes using health information technology tools and patient navigators. J. Diab. Sci. Technol. **6**(1), 169–176 (2012)
103. Freimuth, V.S., Quinn, S.C.: The contributions of health communication to eliminating health disparities. Am. J. Public Health **94**(12), 2053–2055 (2004)

104. Berger, M., Wagner, T.H., Baker, L.C.: Internet use and stigmatized illness. Soc. Sci. Med. **61**(8), 1821–1827 (2005)
105. Heilig, C.M.S.P.: Ethics in Public Health Surveillance. In: Lee, L.M.T.S, Thacker, S.B. (eds.) Oxford University Press, Oxford (2010)
106. Pew Research Center.: Americans' privacy strategies Post-Snowden Washington, D.C. 2015. Retrieved on July 10, 2017. http://www.pewinternet.org/2015/03/16/americans-privacy-strategies-post-snowden/
107. Gostin, L.O., Sapsin, J.W., Teret, S.P., Burris, S., Mair, J.S., Hodge Jr., J.G., Vernick, J.S.: The model state emergency health powers act: planning for and response to bioterrorism and naturally occurring infectious diseases. JAMA **288**(5), 622–628 (2002)

Printed in the United States
By Bookmasters

Printed in the United States
By Bookmasters